C000049758

Detoxing Naturally Diet

Cleanse and detoxify your body with natural foods and drinks, discover the top detoxing tips to maximize the potential benefits.

James Wiedemann

Table of Contents

Chapter 1:

Introduction

A little over a decade ago, if you mentioned the concept of detoxing, people would laugh it off as a sick joke. Today, almost literally everyone is detoxing. More so, everyone has become an 'expert' on matters detoxing. Some of the most selling books and magazines are on detoxing guides. The internet is filled with blogs and articles about the 'best', 'easiest' and 'latest' detox tips. Pharmaceutical industries are making a killing from products believed to boost detoxing which are literally flying off the shelves in drug stores. The world is very toxic and knowing how to lead a healthy lifestyle is necessary. Therefore, creating awareness on health issues and encouraging people to embrace healthy lifestyles is a step in the right direction. You are probably wondering, why is detoxing specifically so popular? I would say it has everything to do with control. There are things in life that we have control over and others that we don't. I believe that we all have control over what goes into our bodies and how we treat our bodies. We don't have control over economies, politics or other external factors, but we are in control of our bodies. We are living in times where there is a lot of information that is mostly contradicting. It leaves as confused and without clear answers on different issues. Some of the issues that we are most concerned about include;

- Minimalism in our homes décor
- Cleaner homes
- Mind health through practices such as yoga and meditation
- Physical health and longevity

Detoxing is just one of the many ways we are trying to achieve a healthier lifestyle. There is a lot of commercial greed in the detoxing industry. A lot has been put out there in form of products and procedures on the best way to detox. It is important to keep in mind that these are just marketing gimmicks. No two people are exactly the same, even twins. Therefore, people will not have the exact same detox experience. The best approach to detoxing is to find out what will work best for your body and lifestyle.

Detoxing and Science

It is ironic that detoxing is so popular yet there is very little scientific evidence on its effectiveness. Therefore, there is no founded prove that detoxing is a cure to any diseases or improves one's health. However, there is a lot of anecdotal evidence spanning over a 100 years. Naturopathy has also advocated for the importance of detoxing. However, the scientific and medical research so far has provided factual information that cannot be ignored. The medical community has discovered that toxins in the body are increasingly leading to chronic diseases. Though this is already proven, it is yet to become a popular base for treatment. Detoxing has health benefits on major organs in the body. These organs are;

- Liver
- Lungs
- Kidneys
- Intestines
- Skin
- Lymphatic system

Types of toxins

- Anti-nutrients; caffeine, alcohol and processed foods
- After products of chemical processes in the body. They include; nitrogen, urea, carbon dioxide, bile and stool
- Abusing medication
- Heavy metals; mercury, arsenic and lead

- Allergens; chemicals, pollen, dust and food
- Bacteria, yeast, viruses and parasites which cause infection
- Chemicals such as herbicides, pesticides and household cleaning detergents.

Social, emotional and spiritual issues which affect our health

- Stressful conditions such as worrying too much, overworking, inadequate rest and financial strain
- Mental issues such as addiction, emotional eating and low self esteem
- Things in the surrounding environment that distract us such as; smells, noises and light
- Being excessively stimulated by radio, computers, television and mobile phones
- Lack of meaning and purpose for your life

- Being isolated, lonely and lacking social support from family, friends and colleagues
- Disconnection with the natural environment
- Having negative emotions and thoughts

Detoxing can be a remedy for improving very serious medical conditions. The paramount importance of liver functions has to be taken as key. Allergies, inflammation and metabolic disorders can gravely affect the functions of the liver. Some of the resulting disorders are; asthma, arthritis, eczema, chronic infections and hormonal imbalance. Physical changes caused by detoxing also have emotional impacts. For example, mood shifts are common during detoxing. The emotional changes can be positive or negative. It is therefore important to expect them and know how best to deal and control them. The emotional impact can be referred to as 'emotional detox'. During the process, old built up emotions resurface. They can take a mental toll on you therefore you are advised to deal with emotional issues prior to detoxing. Detoxing includes eliminating caffeine and alcohol. It helps in balancing your energy levels, giving you mind clarity and focus. If you suffer from insomnia, it will become a thing in the past. Your sleep improves and you are well rested, enabling you perform other functions well. The ideal detox involves elimination diet. Elimination diet is used in diagnosing food sensitivity and intolerance. Therefore detoxing can help you diagnose food intolerance. Medical research on some participants with medical conditions has proven that the conditions improved or were completely eliminated after detoxing. Such medical conditions include; asthma, sinusitis, migraines, chest pains and PMS. On the other hand, food intolerance can cause negative mental effects. The effects can cause one to be; depressed, forgetful, confused, irritable, aggressive and hyperactive. If you suspect you have food intolerance, do not diagnose yourself. Detox under the guidance of a medical professional. This will enable you reintroduce foods which you suspect you are intolerant to, after detoxing. It will help you identify the problematic foods. This can be explained by the types of foods consumed during detoxing. The amounts of food are not limited or restricted while detoxing. However, foods which are notorious for leading to weight gain are limited during detoxing. They include; refined sugar, refined carbs, saturated fats and alcohol. Detoxing helps in creating consistent healthy eating habits. You are able to follow through a healthy weight loss plan. However, detoxing is not a magic wand. It cannot cure underlying serious medical conditions. It may however improve the tolerance to the medical conditions. Those with health issues should seek medical professional guidance. They should also have realistic expectations on what to expect when detoxing. Detoxing is not a miracle major life changes. Only you have the power to turn around your life through consistent good choices. However, detoxing will put you on the right path.

Benefits of the natural detox diet

1. You can forget about ever counting calories or restricting food portions

Conventional dieting is just absolute torture. Most of you might be familiar with the experience. You are restricted from eating tasty food and the amounts of what you eat are ridiculously small. You are literally starving all the time. Hunger causes you to be moody almost all the time. Most of those diets leave you worse off than you were before. A popular misgiving experienced by those trying to lose weight through dieting is instead gaining more weight. A natural detox diet is different. It will involve good healthy food and in satiable amounts. With a natural detox diet, you realize what you have been missing out on. You will be able to happily stick to the diet your whole life.

2. You will eat great amounts on nutrient rich and satisfying foods

Most people follow mainstream diet routines. Majority of these routines are just fads that are targeting a vulnerable society for quick financial gain. They mostly worsen health conditions and may cause ailments. You will therefore realize how fortunate you are to have discovered a natural detox diet. The diet allows you to consume delicious food in wholesome quantities. Some of the delightful foods that are a taboo in dieting are allowed in a natural detox diet. The foods taste great, are filling and most importantly healthy. It is wrong to think that you cannot have all those qualities in one diet, because it is possible.

3. Every area of your life will dramatically improve

Think of the natural detox diet as much more than just what you eat. Think of it as a lifestyle because the program affects how you live. When you embrace the guidance we are offering within this E-book, you are set to improve your life positively. The diet helps you attain a clearer mental state, handle your emotions better and create meaningful emotional connections. Cleansing your body will lead to you cleaning out other areas of your life. You will want to improve your living space so as to reflect and meditate on what is happening within you. You will be inspired to live and communicate better with yourself and others. You will be honest with yourself and get a clear picture of what is going on in your life and your surrounding environment. A deeper understanding of your inner self will boost your confidence. A natural detox diet means you respect your body, to maintain its health. When you respect your body, you respect yourself and others. Your physical health will also improve greatly. You will experience wellness and your health conditions, even those chronic, will improve. You will depend less on medication to treat or minimize the effects of ailments. Your body will be able to cleanse and heal itself. The natural diet detox program greatly enhances your lifestyle in so many ways. It wouldn't be possible to name all of the benefits, since they are so many. Once you experience the good changes that the diet brings, you will never want to turn back to your old ways.

4. You will gain fast results that will improve throughout your lifetime

Detoxifying the body through consumption of natural foods is a way of life. The goal is to detox and maintain the gains in the long-term. You cannot achieve the full benefits of a detox if you go back to your old unhealthy habits after a detox. The program teaches you how to enjoy eating healthy foods so as to constantly improve your diet and maintain your health. A common problem with traditional diets is that nobody wants to follow them long-term. The natural food detox diet starts to work from your first meal. It offers a great living experience so that you desire to make it your permanent regime.

What a Cleanse means

During a cleanse diet, you cut out processed foods such as junk foods, saturated fats, refined carbohydrates, fried foods and animal products. Alcohol is also restricted in this diet. The foods which are eliminated are toxic. You get to feed your body organic foods which are free of chemical additives and preservatives. The foods in the diet are raw and their natural form. This is what your body really needs. There are two methods in which a cleanse works. The first way is when you do not consume traditional foods. It leads to release of toxins to your digestive system. The toxins get trapped in your body system. Some of the areas they can get trapped are in the; blood, tissues, skin and internal organs. The internal organs are very sensitive and some damage may be irreversible. The toxins are a consistent danger through exposure when they are trapped in the body. They can cause; water retention, poor energy, and poor digestion. They can lead to a weak immune system and cause dry hair and scaly skin. Let me paint you a scenario that may be relatable to all of us. You have been hitting the gym every day and doing intense work outs. However, your weight remains the same or in some cases, you actually gain weight. Or you spend weeks on a vacation, eating, drinking and making merry. Most foods you consume during this time are fast foods, junk and alcohol. It is no surprise that your skinny jeans don't fit after the trip. If you continue to eat and drink toxic foods, the problem only worsens. The second method is to eliminate the toxins. In this process, the body focuses its energy in clearing out the system. It doesn't concentrate on digestive processes. An ideal cleanse would include a lot of fiber and nutrients rich food intake. These foods will produce enzymes and antioxidants needed by the body to clear out its system. This E-Book has a great goal. The goal is to help and guide you in detoxing and a pleasant cleanse experience. Some of the topics will delve into how to conduct an easy cleanse regime and what to do after. You will also learn how to manage any detox symptoms that you may experience as a result of the detox programs. The E-book also provides some tasty and healthy recipes to fit into the detox programs meal plans. I know most of you have probably tried cleanse programs that you easily gave up after getting frustrated by the process or starving. You must have been doing it wrong. You will learn the right and easy way to detox and get satisfactory results in the end. The cleanse experience here is different from anything you've heard or read before. The programs here consist of healthy recipes and other practices that give you strength and energy as you lead a healthy and happy lifestyle. Forget about hunger and starvation as you detox. We encourage you to consume raw fruits and vegetables to your fill. We replace your processed unhealthy foods with natural foods. We will encourage you to drink plenty of water for a cleanse experience like no other. If you follow all the steps in the right way, you will have a peaceful and pleasant cleanse experience. You will feel fabulous and be heathier. Best of all, you don't have to break the bank for a successful detox experience. Keeping all this in mind, let's get started!

Chapter 2:

Detoxification and why you need it

Detoxification is a natural process in the body. The body neutralizes and eliminates toxins rom its system, in this process. The body has in-built detox systems. They are the livers and kidneys. However, the body was not meant to handle the chemical laden foods that are now so common in our diets. The body needs to be fed with healthy foods for it to carry out its functions effectively. There is a way that you can avoid conducting cleansing and the body will remain healthy. It is by consuming an organic plant based diet all through. However, is this really possible in today's world and the lifestyles most people lead? The reality is that we are exposed to toxins in the environment every single day we step out. Therefore, the realistic solution is to detox so as to remove the toxins which build up in our digestive systems. It separates fiber and nutrients and passes waste through the colon. On the other hand, the body is unable to separate processed foods. They include; additives, chemicals and fast foods. The body is not able to identify the healthy and non-healthy components of these foods. It leads to build up of toxins in the digestive system. This is because the toxins cannot pass through the colon. The buildup can take weeks, months and even years. This can be a very dangerous risk that may be fatal since the digestive organs may get blocked or eventually fail in performing their functions properly. There are symptoms that may mean that the body's natural detox capability is at risk. For example; if the effects of caffeinated drinks such as tea and coffee take several hours to wear off or cause insomnia, it may be a sign that the liver is not neutralizing toxins effectively. The symptom also applies if you have high sensitivity to smells such as perfumes and chemicals. Other common symptoms of the detox system's imbalance include;

- **Slow lymphatic system**: Its symptoms are; frequent colds, cellulite, fatigue and puffy eyes
- **Overload in the liver**: Bloating, feeling nauseated and indigestion
- **Congestion in the lungs**: running nose, blocked sinuses and frequent sneezing
- **Stressed kidneys**: Observe your urine for the following; dark-colored, scanty, cloudy and strong smell. Also if you experience pain when you urinate
- **Overly stretched out skin**: cellulite, pimples, rashes, blackheads and whiteheads
- **Toxins in the intestines**: constipation and migraines

If you experience at least three of the following symptoms, you should consider a detoxing. If you experience most of the symptoms, consult a medical practitioner.

Detoxing the right way

There is a craze for fasting and cleansing as the ultimate way to achieve successful detoxing results. Many people are falling for the hype but the claims on the results are not factual. Here, you will learn how to separate the hype from reality. For many years, there has been unending debate on the benefits and risks of detoxing. Medical professionals have forwarded a strong argument that the body can detoxify itself. This is because the body has a highly effective system for eliminating waste and toxins. Both arguments have solid points. It is true that the body has a very complex and highly effective in-built detoxification system. The major organs for the detoxification process are; liver, lungs, kidneys, intestines and skin. The functions of these major organs are as follows;

- **Liver**: Traps toxins circulating in the blood stream
- **Kidneys**: clear out by-products of digestion and the build-up of minerals. The by-products include uric acid
- **Lungs**: They conduct filtration of the air we inhale and expel toxic air through exhalation
- **Skin**: Removes toxins through sweat
- **Intestines**: Contain bacteria which neutralizes toxins before eliminating food waste

The body may not always be able to handle detoxification that we subject it to. The body responds well to early preventive measures as compared to late intervention. Conventional medicine is a solution to toxins only when the body is at risk of complete shutdown. An example is kidney dialysis. It is a process whereby toxic elements are removed from the blood. This is in the event of kidney failure, where kidneys cannot perform this function of blood filtration. There has been controversial claims that healthy people expose themselves to unnecessary danger by detoxing. However, health professionals have pointed out that body organs give warning signs before complete failure or shutdown. The body organs give these warning signs through overload and stress. We come across a number of environmental and food toxins every day. We should work to strengthen and support the natural detoxification system of the body. It would be the most realistic and safe measure to take in preserving our body's detoxification systems. It helps the body avoid the risk of health conditions with time and age. It also boosts good health and longevity. A good detox program can be a great boost to your overall wellbeing since it enhances your physical, mental and spiritual wellbeing. There are many people who are caught in the middle, in the detoxing fanfare. They do want to get rid of unwanted toxins. At the same time, they do not know the safest and healthiest detox programs to follow. It's good to note that some detox programs are unhealthy and may end up doing more harm than good. The body is built to handle certain levels of toxins. The problem comes in when there is excessive intake or production of toxins. Reduced rate of eliminating toxins is also a major problem since it can lead to overloading of the body system. Such problems in elimination of toxins are the primary cause of chronic health conditions. The conditions include; headaches, digestive problems, overweight and confused thinking. The current culture and societal has made it difficult for the physical body to keep up. The modern lifestyle has exposed us to an increasingly toxic environment. In this regard, the detoxification body systems are overworked. They have to work overtime to process, neutralize and eliminate the toxins that we come across in our day to day lives. Some of the systems have been worked way past their capacity and capabilities. The situation leads to detoxing elimination systems requiring artificial support to function properly. Let us learn how to maintain our body systems healthy without overloading them. After all, we have only one body that cannot be replaced.

Be warned of the dangerous quick fix

In 2006, celebrity musician and actress Beyoncé Knowles lost twenty pounds in two weeks. The drastic change was for a movie role. There was a lot of internet talk and speculation that the weight loss was achieved through a detox program. She claimed to have used a lemon water fast. The fast was known as "Master cleanse". The Master cleanse gained popularity among people who wanted to achieve fast weight loss. Health professionals discourage using such detox programs to lose weight. Such programs are mostly ineffective and counterproductive. Use of extreme detox programs such as fasts should be avoided. If one has to undertake such a detox, it should be with the guidance of a medical or health practitioner. Medical experts recommend moderate detoxing with whole natural foods. The detox foods should be accompanied by nutritional supplements. Benefits of nutritional supplements include;

- They are safe
- They have more and actual health benefits
- Less likelihood for them to negatively affect metabolic processes
- They do not cause weight gain

Detox programs have health benefits when practiced in a healthy way. They also help in improving vitality. Also, people who detox are able to adopt healthier eating habits. This helps them achieve sustainable weight loss, which is the goal for most people who detox. It is surprising that the quick fix regimes are more popular yet they are unsustainable. Most spas and salons have footbath treatments that are claimed to remove toxins through the feet. There are body wraps which are advertised as able to shrink off body weight and fat. Cleansing kits with promises of fast successful results are fast selling. Fast weight loss is a very attractive notion that is guaranteed to attract consumers who are conscious of their body weight and appearance. This has made some detox programs irresistible to consumers. Detoxing and fasting specifically to achieve weight loss is a new concept. It is also not a healthy strategy, according to health experts. Fasting is a historic culture. People have always fasted with the main aim being wellbeing and sometimes for spiritual purposes. No historic evidence points out at fasting as a remedy to achieve weight loss. We should have a more open minded outlook on detoxing the body. Healthy detoxing is about improving physical and emotional wellbeing. It should not be focused on weight loss or finding miraculous cures for chronic illnesses. All the hype and attractive promises of detoxing have created unrealistic expectations. Extreme detoxing may seem attractive as a way of achieving fast results, but it is highly dangerous. Anything that promises almost instant results is most likely untrue. Healthy detoxing involves meal plans and a time frame for the achievements to kick in. it is realistic and requires you to put in effort, commitment and dedication. Healthy detoxification will heal your body and improve how you feel.

Who is meant to detox?

In the toxic environment we all live in, detoxing would be good for everyone. However, not everyone can undergo the elimination in detox programs. If a person has symptoms such as pale and puffy skin or discoloration in the eyes, they should not start a detox program. It could be a recipe for trouble further down the road. The person should take nutrient supplements and fiber in their diet to improve their condition. It is ironic that those who are most depleted to start a detox program are the ones who require it most. Your body system may be overloaded with years of excessive exposure to toxins. The condition may be as a result of consuming processed foods, emotional eating or going through chronic stress. If a person experiences such conditions, they should consider a supervised detox. The supervised detox involves meeting with nutrition professionals at least once or twice a week. The guidance from the professional will ensure you get the right amount of nutrition and hydration you need as your body undergoes the healing process. People who suffer digestive diseases should be supervised. The digestive diseases include; colitis and diverticulitis. The insoluble fiber supplements used in detox programs can worsen these conditions. People with eating disorders should also seek professional guidance. Fasting when you have an eating disorder can negatively affect your emotional balance. For most people who are generally healthy, mild detox programs which don't require supervision have many health benefits. There are a few symptoms which might be an indication that your body is not processing toxins as it should. They include; migraines, low energy, bloating and breaking of the skin. There are some detoxes which can help the situation. They include; increasing nutrient and fiber in your food and eliminating processed foods from your diet. These are just mild interventions that anyone can easily incorporate. There are other intense interventions such as fasting with juice or broth. The intense interventions should however be brief since they cannot sustain the body needs over a long period of time.

The right detox will be dependent on your health, availability and the problems you want a solution to. For a proper detox experience, you should individualize the program. You should also be focused, determined and committed to achieving your goals through the detox program. When you put all these into perspective, it helps your intentions be revealed clearly and healthily. Your detox journey will be guided by passion rather than fear. If the major goal is weight loss, do not jump into the fast bandwagon of detox programs being used by celebrities. It will most likely not work. They are most likely just endorsements to sell products and promote brands. Fasting is a very temporary measure for achieving weight loss. You are very likely to overeat after the fast period therefore your gains are erased. This is because the body stores toxins in fat to provide protection to vital internal organs. This is a reaction to when the body is unable to effectively eliminate toxins. If you want to maintain weight loss, the best bet is by making lifestyle changes. This is the healthiest and most effective solution. You should adopt new dieting habits which are healthy. They should consist whole natural foods.

The best time to cleanse

Each person has different detox needs. However, the recommended general advice is having a three to six days detox quarterly. That means four times in a year, preferably every three months. So how will you know when it's time to detox? When you experience the most common symptoms such as feeling fatigued or bloated, you can result to a light cleanse. The experience will help your body system reset for better functioning. You can use natural fibers and water to help clear up toxins and waste buildup in the colon. Restrict your diet from processed foods, refined sugars and salt and saturated fats. When you remove these foods from your diet, the body releases the toxins that had built up. Such foods include raw fruits and vegetables. When the body releases toxins, probiotics help in restoring the balance of bacteria in the digestive system. The modern world has very many toxins that can imbalance our digestive systems. This makes it very difficult to maintain digestive health. Short term cleanses provides the digestive system with an opportunity for recovery from toxins. The digestive system is able to heal itself.

Detoxing for weight loss

The world today is obsessive with quick fixes for everything, especially weight loss. Therefore, you should be wise by reviewing any quick fix solutions with skepticism. The plan we offer here will help you lose weight. However, it is not designed solely for the purpose of weight loss. The main aim of the program is guide you in experimenting with your body to find out what works for you and what doesn't. Through the program, you will immediately realize how better you look and feel by consuming whole natural foods. The results may be seen in just a single week. Follow through the program for seven days consistently. You will experience benefits such as; reduced inflammations and less toxin buildup. The end result will be slimming of your face and body. Other benefits will be; better sleep patterns, increased energy, glowing healthy skin, reduced pain in the joints and better elimination. Chronic discomfort also reduces significantly. Such benefits should encourage you to adopt a healthy lifestyle of consuming healthy foods. A healthy lifestyle will help you maintain your ideal weight and increased vitality easily. Research and decades of medical observation have determined that the things that make people sick are the same things that contribute to weight gain. Resolving health conditions such as inflammation and toxicity also contributes to weight loss. There is a common factor between chronically overweight patients. When they adopt healthy eating habits and realize it is actually working, they are motivated to make healthy lifestyle changes. A one week detox experience helps you realize that you have the power to harm or heal your body. You realize that consuming bad foods make you sick and on the other hand, healthy foods help you maintain your ideal weight and boost your health. People under medication should consult medical practitioners before undertaking a detox program. In this program, you are provided with a meal plan that specifies what to eat and when to eat it. You will lose weight but at the same time gain much needed energy.

Preparation for the detox program

A week before starting the detox program, you need to prepare your body for what to expect. There is a lot of good to expect from getting rid of habits that negatively affect your metabolism. Eliminating unhealthy foods from your diet systematically prevents withdrawal symptoms. It also helps you begin the journey to ideal weight and good health. During the week of preparation, you should completely remove these components from your diet. In some cases, the toxins may be hidden in a way that is not easily detectable. When buying food stuffs, check the label for the contents. Ensure you entirely avoid the following foods;

- Caffeine. Only green tea is permissible
- Refined carbohydrates
- Refined sugar
- Trans-fats

- Processed junk foods
- Fast foods
- Alcohol

When the preparation week is over, you can begin the seven day sliming program. We have given you different recipes in this E-book to use for daily meal plans. Ensure the meals are well balanced and nutrient rich. Spare sometime every day to prepare foods and beverages you will require daily to carry to work or consume in your day to day activities. Some recipes are for foods which can be prepared in advance and refrigerated, for example broth. However, other foods and beverages should be prepared just before consuming. During the first two days, your energy may decrease. You may experience low energy during the first two days. If this happens, you should rest and take time to heal yourself. Get enough sleep, go to a spa and get a body massage. All this will help your body recover and heal. Cleansing can help in weight loss programs.

If you want the weight loss to be short term, use high fiber and nutrient rich diets to lose weight in a healthy way. You will look and feel slimmer and healthier. You feel good about your body and appearance. In America, women get an approximate 50% of the daily serving recommended for fiber. Men get approximately 40% of the recommended amount. This percentages may be low as a result of ignorance or the type of lifestyle common in the West. Most of the foods consumed on a daily basis are fast foods that have low or no fiber content. Fiber helps us feel full after eating even without consuming a lot. It expands the digestive system and helps us feel full for long. Feeling full prevents one from overeating. High fiber consumption eases the digestion and bowel movement processes. Soluble fibers help in lowering blood cholesterol. This is done by preventing excessive absorption of cholesterol in the diet and lowering blood sugar levels. Dietary fiber protects against high C-reactive protein, popularly known as CRP. CRP is one of the leading causes of cardiovascular diseases. Cleansing is also a good source of hydration. This is because it involves intake of high amounts of water, regularly. When you drink water, you avoid high sugar intake. Beverages with high calorie content are the major sources of sugar. When you consume water, your thirst is satisfied therefore you don't require to consume sugary beverages. Water also helps clear out excess salts that cause bloating and constipation. The body weight is approximately 60% water. Therefore, it is very important in major body functions and the general health of the body system. Efficient hydration helps the body transport nutrients and flush out toxins. One of the major organs that is highly dependent on adequate water in the body, is the kidneys. The kidneys regulate fluid balance and flow in the body. They function well when the water supply is efficient. If the kidneys don't receive enough water, they produce concentrated urine. These means they utilize more energy leading to wearing out of tissues. This may happen when the kidneys are stressed. Kidneys are under stress when the foods you consume contain very high amounts of salt or other toxins that have to be cleared out. When you drink enough water, the salt or toxins are diluted, thus protecting the kidneys. Dehydration can cause negative effects on cognitive performance. These effects include; improper digestion and headaches. When you are undertake a detox or cleanse program ensure you are well hydrated all through. Proper hydration will ensure body systems function properly and reduce the possibility of experiencing detox side effects. Eliminating toxic foods from your diet also eliminates the craving for these foods. When you identify the cause of your cravings, for example medical treatment, you should change your diet habits to minimize the cravings. If you want to avoid cravings, you should consume a healthy protein in your meals. It will help in maintaining your blood sugar at healthy levels, while at the same time promoting satiety.

Simple slim down program

The program is conducted within seven days. Here are the foods that are recommended for the program.

- At least 6-8 glasses of water per day
- Fish. The most highly recommended are sardines, sole, herring, black cod, cod and wild salmon.
- Organic lean white meat such as chicken breasts
- Organic non-citrus fruits such as berries. They can be fresh or frozen
- Organic fresh vegetables
- At least 3 cups of vegetable broth a day
- Legumes such as kidney beans

- Organic lemons
- Organic ground flaxseeds

There are foods that you should avoid during the program. Most of these foods are inflammatory and full of toxins. Some of the foods listed may not be problematic to you. However, the best way to find out is eliminate them for a week and observe if there are any changes in your body. These foods are;

- Sugar products increases mood swings and fogs brain memory. It also destroys good bacteria, thus slowing down the process of detoxification.
- Sugar alcohols such as xylitol, sorbitol and maltitol
- Dairy products such as milk, cheese and butter. Dairy has an acidic effect to the body. It causes cells to function poorly and also slows down the detox process.
- Corn

- Meat such as beef, pork and lamb. Organic poultry is an allowed exception. Meat slows down digestion. It also blocks bowels and causes breeding of bacteria in your guts.
- Flour and flour products
- Artificial sweeteners such as aspartame
- Yeast and fermented foods
- Eggs
- Alcohol. It causes toxicity to the liver. It also decreases the amounts of magnesium and zinc which are required in the detoxification process.
- Gluten in wheat products. Wheat causes poor nutrient intake. It also causes irritation of the intestines' lining. It also leads to bloating, constipation and indigestion.
- Caffeine (except green tea). It leads to an increase in toxins in the body.

- Processed foods. They contain high levels of sugar, salt and bad fats. High salt content is bad for blood pressure
- Citrus fruits and juices
- Natural sweeteners such as stevia
- Food additives. Most of these are made from petrochemicals. They release toxins to the liver and make the process of detoxification very difficult.
- Packaged foods containing chemicals
- Peanuts
- Night shades such as bell peppers and tomatoes
- Refined oils and other bad fats. They cause the liver to strain in its function
- Stimulants such as diet pills

Simple meal plan

A simple meal plan should eliminate the foods that we have recommended you to eliminate and incorporate the recommended foods. When you do this, your body is nourished and healthy. Your metabolism will greatly improve over the seven days period. The program does not leave you feeling physically hungry, unlike most detox programs. There are recommended bath treatments that help your body release toxins and leave you rejuvenated. Here is a simple meal plan for a day in this program.

Breakfast: 7 a.m. to 9 a.m.

- ½ a lemon squeezed in hot water
- A cup of green tea

You should take a maximum of two cups of green tea in a day. You should expect bowel movement by 10 a.m. If it doesn't occur naturally, take two herbal laxative tablets

- A cup of green tea

Lunch 12 p.m. to 1 p.m.

- Two cups of lightly sautéed vegetables
- ½ a cup of brown rice
- ½ a cup of fruit
- ounces of chicken breast

- 5 ounces of tofu
- 2 cups of steamed veggies
- ½ a cup of brown rice
- A cup of broth

Broth Recipe

The modern diet produces acid. It includes sugars, excessive animal proteins and processed foods. They create a toxic cellular environment that can lead to diseases. The broth recipe provided has many healing nutrients. It is a good way of detoxification and alkalinizing the body. The recipe is as follows

- ½ cup seaweed
- A cup of daikon, largely cubed
- 2 stalks of celery, cubed
- A cup of root vegetables such as turnips, largely cubed
- ½ cup of cabbage
- 2 cups of chopped greens such as dandelion, kale and parsley
- 4 ½ inch of knob ginger

- A cup of fresh mushrooms (optional)

Add enough water to cover. Place to boil over low heat for an hour. After it boils, simmer to taste. Drink at least 3 cups a day.

Shake recipe

This recipe provides essential proteins. The proteins help in detoxification, provide fiber for better digestion and increase elimination from flaxseeds. It is easy to make and digest. You can eat raw veggies as alternative snacks.

- 2 scoops of rice
- Ice (optional)
- Water
- non-citrus organic fruits. They include blueberries, strawberries, cherries, bananas and pears.
- 1 tbsp. nut butter (optional). The nuts can be; almond, macadamia or pecan
- A cup of combined nuts such as almonds, walnuts and pecans

Digestion

The best thing to eliminate from your diet during a detox is gluten. Gluten is majorly found in wheat and wheat products. There is a new condition that has been discovered by medical researchers, known as 'Leaky Gut'. It contributes greatly to autoimmune diseases. The condition is explained as follows; there is a barrier in the intestines. The barrier determines whether our bodies can withstand toxic substances or whether they react negatively to toxins. The toxins are mostly those which we are exposed to in the environment. Breaching of the barrier can only occur if one has a 'leaky gut'. It is caused by toxic substances in food such as gluten and chemicals. Such chemicals include; arsenic and BPA. The chemicals cause an immune response in the body which affects the gut, internal organs and tissues. These organs include; the skeleton, pancreas, liver, kidney and brain. Gluten causes damage to the intestines, making them leaky. A leaky gut leads to several medical conditions. The conditions include; obesity and diabetes. Autoimmune disease can also be caused by a leaky gut. Apart from consuming high fiber content, there are other benefits for digestion. There are other natural aids in digestion such as; ginger enzymes and magnesium. Water is also key in ensuring smooth digestion. Physical activities increase the rate of digestion. Physical activity leads to increase of blood flow in the body organs. It also enhances muscle function and helps the internal organs function more efficiently. Probiotic culture is also useful in digestion. Probiotics are good bacteria. They are naturally found in the body and help in keeping the intestines in healthy condition and help in bowel movement.

Why you should avoid animal products during a detox

Detoxing removes fats, nitrates and animal based bacteria from the digestive system. This is a very significant benefit. The best way to do this is eliminate all animal products from your diet during detox. If you are so used to these products, remember that this is just a short term measure. The short time span you eliminate these foods will allow the body to get rid of toxins that have built up in the body. The toxins may have been consumed by eating animal products. Such toxins are; hormones, bacteria, antibiotics and steroids.

Why you should avoid dairy products during a detox

There are people who are intolerant to dairy products. Infants have enzymes that helps them digest dairy products. This is why most babies enjoy milk, including breast milk. With age, we lose these enzymes therefore our bodies find it more difficult to process and digest dairy. There are people who completely abstain from dairy. Others supplement dairy intake with enzyme pills. The intolerance to dairy is known as inflammation. Inflammation can cause bloating, weight gain, digestive problems and allergies. It can also cause mucus congestion and poor skin and hair. When you conduct a short term detox, eliminate dairy. This is a good measure to ensure reduced inflammation. You will have to forego smoothies and shakes since most have a dairy element such as milk.

Why you need a sustainable detox program

The world is changing rapidly. People's behaviors and cultures are also changing.

Climate change has become one of the biggest concerns for mankind today. It affects every human being and will affect every generation to come. Therefore, we have a moral obligation to ensure we leave a healthy planet for future generations. We can only do this by ensuring we address the climate change issue and how to mitigate the effects for a better future. One of the major ways to address climate change is by looking at what is in our plates. Where does the foods you consume come from? Food should not travel thousands of miles to reach a consumer. This is because outsourcing food from far leaves behind a large carbon footprint, for example the carbon emitted by cargo plans and trucks as they transport the foods. We should embrace locally produced foods and consume them raw and natural. Processing of foods also contributes to global warming since manufacturing processes include emission of toxic gases, by-products and wastes to the environment. This directly translates to a more toxic environment, hence global warming which leads to climate change. Other factors to consider is the storage of foods. When we store foods, we utilize a lot of energy in terms of refrigeration. Eating fresh foods is good for your health and helps in reducing the carbon footprint left behind by refrigeration. The best way to reduce your carbon footprint is by eliminating animal products from your diet. Some of the industries with the largest demand and carbon footprint are the meat and dairy industries. They use fossil fuels, destroy and pollute land in their activities. Cow flatulence is also a leading contributor to carbon footprint. According to the United Nations, there is a large production of carbon through meat production. Meat production makes up about 22% of the total greenhouse gases produced globally, annually. That is a very large percentage that should concern everyone. If we all take personal responsibility, that figure can drastically reduce. Beef production releases more greenhouse gases than producing potatoes. Why then not choose the healthier plant option? The consumer has absolute power in deciding what they choose to consume. They should therefore be encouraged to choose other options which have less effects on the climate, as opposed to animal products. Detox should be kind to your body and to your planet. You have only one of both. Your detox should also be kind to animals. If you want to lead a healthy and happy life, you must embrace your role in this world. Don't consume animal products, even for just three days. Notice how your soul and body will be cleansed. It will help you make lifestyle decisions such as completely eliminating animal products from your diet.

Who shouldn't detox?

Detoxing is not for everyone. The detox program is restricts calorie intake therefore it cannot be recommended for some groups of people.

If you are under medication, dealing with a health issue or suffer from underlying and chronic ailments, you should seek the guidance of a medical professional before undertaking a detox program. Additionally, you should not consume foods you are allergic to or are sensitive to. You also don't have to eat foods that you dislike. If you are recovering from eating disorder, alcohol abuse or drug addiction, you should not detox unless under the guidance of a medical professional.

Chapter 3:

How to conduct a healthy detox

It comes as a surprise to most first time detoxes when people realize their bodies have to ease into and out of the process. Your body needs to be tuned to the process by allowing it enough time to adjust. An example is how you prepare for exercise by stretching out your body to tune it to the activities you are about to carry out. We should look forward to making our detox experiences as pleasant and comfortable as possible. Therefore, we should give the body time to ease in since it will allow you to be more comfortable. When the body is at ease, you are less likely to experience the uncomfortable detox symptoms which mostly show at the beginning of the detox program. Many people use the last day before a detox in an unhealthy way. They consume a lot of junk foods since they figure they are about to detox the body system. The practice is not good. If you consume junk foods just before a detox, you may experience most detox symptoms and side effects. This is because your body is suddenly thrown off balance by having to flush out the high amounts of toxins you ingested. The same applies to alcohol consumption. Do not go all in by eliminating everything at once when detoxing. Start by removing animal products, junk, processed and refined foods from your diet. Heavy oils and salty foods can be eliminated after two to three days before you begin detoxing. As you eliminate these foods, introduce raw whole foods, fruits and vegetables in your diet. Those components will help your body detox naturally, easily and healthily. It's all about replacing the foods you eat with healthier options. Instead of eating beef for your protein intake, go for beans instead. Instead of bread or doughnuts for breakfast, have a fruit bowl. Instead of a hamburger for a mid-day snack, have a veggies broth. During your detox, you should reduce your caffeine intake and eventually eliminate it. Caffeine is a drug that you can be addicted to. When you eliminate it, you are likely to experience withdrawal symptoms such as headaches. The symptoms are as a result of your body's reliability on the adrenal glands to enable bowel movements. If you eliminate caffeine and introduce high fiber intake, you will experience other symptoms. They include; bloating, constipation and headaches. Before the detox program, you can start consuming green tea as a replacement to other caffeinated drinks such as coffee. Organic green tea has very many health benefits.

Top choice a detox platform

You can fast for between twelve hours to seven days. In the most pure fasts, only water is consumed. There are a lot of psychological changes experienced during the process. They include; metabolism effects such as changes in levels of amino acids, hormones and minerals. Periodic fasting is beneficial for some health conditions. Such conditions include; asthma, colitis and sinusitis. You should consult a medical practitioner before, during and after a fast period. People with cancer and neurological disorders are advised against fasting. Limited fasts involve drinking just fruit or veggie juices. Mono-diets are also in the category of limited fasts. It involves restricting your diet to a specific food, but only for a short period of time. Both types of fasts can saturate the system with the nutrients composing the food. It has been used to control obesity and cardiovascular diseases. The grapefruit and cabbage soup diets are fad diets since they promise almost instant weight loss. When you undergo these fasts, you will lose weight but only for a limited amount of time. Therefore, limited fasts and mono-diets are not sustainable weight loss methods. They are also not safe. Detox experts advise against restricted fasts. Limited detox diet utilizes a low toxin diet and has many nutrients that help the body to detox easily. The detox involves eliminating foods and beverages which stress your detox system. The foods are replaced with healthy neutral foods which help in the detoxification process. The process will involve eliminating the following from your diet;

- Caffeine
- Dairy
- Sugar
- Salt
- Processed foods
- Saturated fats

However, nutritional experts and naturopaths have different views regarding animal protein. Naturopaths argue that animal protein should not be incorporated into the detox program. They argue that including animal protein will overwork the liver and kidneys. However, nutritional experts argue that animal protein should be included since the liver requires amino acids which is derived from protein so as to detox. You are the only person who can decide which argument to go with. However, if you have underlying medical issues, you should seek supervision from a qualified physician. The physician will be able to offer guidance on the best detox, fasting and mono-diet that suits you. The process will still have to be carried out under the supervision of a physician. We would recommend a gentle limited detox diet which we have provided in this E-book. This detox helps you maintain ideal energy levels. Limited detox diets should last a maximum of four weeks and ideally less. This is because eliminating some foods from your diet may cause intolerance in the long run.

The levels of detoxification

There are three levels of detoxing which are; strong, medium and mild. You should begin with a mild detox then progress to a stronger detox. Your body requires time to adjust gradually to cleansing. Your liver and bowels should be in good condition so as to get rid of toxins in the body. While detoxing you will experience symptoms. The symptoms will indicate whether the detox is too strong or too mild. You are likely to experience headaches, nausea, body aches and pains. If the symptoms are severe or last for several days, the detox is too strong for you. The next step of action should be to moderate your diet and reducing your supplement intake. During a detox, you are likely to experience more frequent and lose bowel movements. If this happens, it is a good sign that toxins are being eliminated from the body. Reduce magnesium intake if you experience diarrhea. If you constipate, consume more flax seeds.

The process of detoxification

There are always toxins stored in the body at any given time. Experts refer to these toxins as 'body burden'. When the total body burden surpasses a level, body organs that eliminate toxins slowdown in their functioning. A good example is how a water filter that hasn't been changed for some time behaves. Detoxing replenishes nutrients in the body. It also removes toxins that have built up in the body which may affect the working of the body system. A toxins is a substance that irritates or causes harm to the body. There are many sources of toxins in the body. Toxins stress the biochemical and functions of vital organs such as liver, lungs and kidneys. Toxins include airborne pollutants such as diesel fumes and synthetic cleaning products. Substances such as refined sugar and caffeine cause inflammation. Gluten and dairy products are common allergens. Eliminating toxic foods from your diet is helpful in ensuring your body gets rid of toxins efficiently. Take a break from refined sugar, dairy products and caffeine for some weeks. It is not only what you eliminate from your diet that counts, but also what you incorporate in the diet. A good example is fiber. Past generations in America consumed about 30 grams a day. Currently, less than 12 grams of fiber is consumed by people America in a day. This means that the food we eat in a day can be stored in the colon for even a week. Detox programs aim to flush out this toxin buildups in the body organs. There are off-the-shelf detox kits that can do the trick. They contain both soluble and insoluble fiber. They also contain chelating substances which absorb heavy metals. A popular chelating substance used in detox kits is bentonite clay. High quality detox kits are recommended for people who have very busy schedules. These group of people may not have the time to determine the daily dose of clay and fiber that they require to consume. However, for those with the time, you can purchase these substances in bulk at a cheaper cost. An eleven day detox program is recommended in using these substances. During the period, set out the first seven days to consume whole foods which are not allergens. Have a juice fast for one day. The remaining three last days should be used for recovery. Consume probiotic foods during the recovery period. Patients should follow a program that gets rid of allergen foods. The program should also include supplements and salt baths. Yoga is also a good exercise for a great detox experience. The duration of the program is different between people. It's length and frequency is dependent on an individual's needs. Preparation is important before starting a detox program. Some of the things you may prepare for are restoration of nutrients, buildup of organ capacity or to wean the body from processed foods. Preparation is also required when easing back into a detox program. To achieve the full benefits of a detox, you should resume regular eating at a slow pace. This gives your body enough time to adjust to the changes. Experts' advice that one should expect detox side effects in most of the scenarios. It can be as a result of the huge amount of toxins being released into the bloodstream which can cause nausea and headaches. It can also be a result of the elimination of substances such as caffeine and sugar which cause withdrawal symptoms. There are detox symptoms which can show that the process is effective. They include, fatigue, migraines and irritation. Additional symptoms are bad breath, body odor and skin break outs. The symptoms disappear after the first few days of detoxing. The disappearance is enhanced by the continuous release of toxins in the body as it reaches climax.

Day to day detox

A planned detox program may affect your daily routine especially for first timers. It therefore may not be ideal for people with busy schedules or low energy levels. A detox doesn't mean you have to stop everything you do on a daily basis for the process to be effective. You can also receive benefits from the following detox habits;

- **Drinking plenty of water**. Hydration is the best way to help your body eliminate toxins. The kidneys function is to remove waste from the body. They require adequate amount of water to carry out their function. They flush out waste from protein metabolism such as uric acid, urea and lactic acid. We excrete a lot of water through sweating, urinating and breathing. Therefore, we need to consume a lot of water to make up for these loses.

- **Consume organic vegetables**. Adequate fiber content is key in detoxification. The fiber can be obtained from organic vegetables such as kale, parsley, collard greens and cabbage. People who detox are advised to eliminate refined foods and allergens from their diet. They should consume whole, natural foods. Vegetarian diets have multiple detoxification benefits. The diets adds fiber intake and reduces consumption of toxins. Vegetarian diets are also very easy to prepare. Vegetarian diet reduces the amounts of saturated fats, nitrates, antibiotics and hormones you consume. This allows the body to clear out toxins and increase nutrients and antioxidants. There is a detox program known as 'fast track' which includes lean animal protein. Though recommended, one should strictly stick to pasture-raised meat, dairy products and eggs. This will avoid antibiotic and hormonal by-products.

- **Skin scrubs and saunas**. The skin is a major organ in excreting wastes and toxins. Skin scrubs and sauna baths can enhance the process. You can detox your body through skin brushing every day. All you require is a skin brush. The brush should be long with a long handle and coarse bristles. The brush can be found in most food stores which sell natural foods. Brushing the skin helps in removal of toxins from the skins surface. It also improves circulation of blood and lymph. The best way to brush the skin is from outward towards the heart. This particular movement helps lymph fluid to flow in the right direction. The movement also supports vascular valve functions. Sauna baths are also a great way to remove toxins through the skin. For an ultimate experience and to enjoy effective benefits, spend 35 minutes in a sauna. The moderate heat should be around 140 degrees. Most gym sauna set there temperatures at between 185 and 190 degrees. These temperatures may be a bit high therefore you should take a shorter period of time.

- **Probiotics**. In an ideal situation, the bacteria in the colon neutralizes and excretes toxins from the body. Therefore, these bacteria requires a lot of support. There are always supplements which help your flora thrive and be happy. They include; live culture, yogurt, kefir and probiotic supplements.

- **Garlic and cilantro**. Consuming garlic daily removes heavy metals from the body. Garlic has chemical compounds which attract heavy metals. Heavy metals come out of soft tissues and join the sulfur component found in garlic. If your stomach can tolerate, eat your garlic raw. Raw garlic is also very effective in providing a quick solution for detoxification. For a long time effect, consume at least two cloves of garlic daily, to keep heavy metals away. That will work if you want fast detox results. For a daily routine, you can use two cloves of sautéed garlic. It will help keep away heavy metals from your body system. Cilantro has been proven to contain some medicinal properties. It helps in removing mercury from the body. It also has antibacterial and anti-inflammatory properties.

- **Breathe deeply**. Deep breathing helps in removing toxins from the body. It stimulates the nervous system and helps you calm down. This results to a reduction in the buildup of adrenal stress hormones. It also leads to exhalation of toxins. When we are stressed, we breathe shallowly. When this happens, it prevents the regular release of toxins through breathing. Therefore, deep breaths are very essential in releasing toxins from the body. A good detox program is the best way of removing toxins from the body. You should detox for vitality. Control and purity should not be your main goal. When you detox the right way, you will be healthy and happy.

Seven day detox plan

The best time to begin a detox program is during the weekend. Make sure that you do not have a lot of social engagements the following week. This will allow your body enough time to recover from the detox without interruptions. Buy all the foods and supplements you will require for your meal plans in advance. Let your friends and family know that you are detoxing, so that they plan their meals to accommodate your detox, without unnecessary temptations. For the program we offer you, you can consume what suits you best. You can consume three solid meals in a day. You can also opt for small snacks at regular intervals all through the day. The snacks are meant to boost your energy levels. Stick to the foods in your diet plan. Such components in food release toxins in the body which are harmful for your health. Healthy foods contain antioxidants, vitamins and minerals. All these activate the body and help it in its functions. Cells, liver and bowels are aided in their functions by a healthy, natural diet.

Eat abundantly

Organic fruits

- Apricots
- Lemons

- Pawpaw
- Peaches
- Melons
- Berries
- Mangoes
- Kiwi
- Grapes

These organic fruits have alkaline content. They have high antioxidant content. They also contain an amino acid known as 'glutathione'. All these components enhance liver functions and metabolic processes. Melons are diuretic. They have a strong alkalizing effect on the body system. However, do not consume grapefruit or its juice. It contains naringenin. Naringenin can affect the functions of liver enzymes which are utilized in the detox process.

Organic Vegetables

- Artichokes
- Beets
- Green veggies

- Carrots
- Pumpkins
- Watercress
- Bean sprouts
- Capsicums
- Broccoli
- Cucumber
- Cauliflower
- Sweet potatoes

All the above vegetables have an alkalizing effect. They also have high contents of fiber, antioxidants and minerals. Artichokes contain caffeoylquinic acids. These are plant compounds which increase the rate of bile flow and helps in digestion. Generally, vegetables contain enzymes which aid digestion and help in detoxification. Their high fiber content helps in bowel movement.

Eat in moderation

There are foods which enhance the detox process. They include;

- You should consume a maximum portion of portions in a day
- **Fish**; Consume small fish types such as; tilapia, wild salmon, sardines and monkfish. Those type of fish reduce inflammation and boost cell immunity. Remember that the seas and lakes are very contaminated with high metals and other toxic substances which are consumed by fish. Large fish such as tuna and swordfish may be contaminated. Eat fish after the first three days of the detox program.
- You can pick among the variety of almonds, pumpkin seeds, flax seeds, hazelnuts and sunflower seeds. However, avoid them if you are allergic. They contain fat soluble vitamins. The vitamins activate brain cells and enhance cells functioning.
- **Oils**; for cooking, use organic extra virgin oil. It is a healthier replacement for butter or margarine. To dress

salads, use seed oils which are cold-pressed.

- **Potatoes and bananas**: they both increase glucose levels in the blood stream. Consume just one portion in a day.

Hydrate

Water is very important in the digestive system. It helps to excrete wastes and toxins. You should drink a minimum of eight glasses of water per day. Ensure the water is either filtered, bottled or sourced at a spring. Sip the water slowly throughout the day. Do not drink water with your meals since this can dilute the juices that aid digestion. For hot beverages, take green tea, herb tea or dandelion coffee. Dandelion is a great liver tonic and has benefits for the digestive system. The beverages are very healthy alternatives to caffeine. They help you detox and maintain a healthy balanced body system.

Foods you should avoid

- Meat
- Eggs
- Wheat products
- Dairy products such as milk, cheese and butter
- Salt
- Processed and refined foods
- Saturated fats
- Fast foods
- Sugary snacks such as cakes and cookies
- Additives and preservatives
- Artificial sweeteners
- Alcohol
- Caffeine
- Carbonated drinks such as soda
- Hydrogenated fats

Infusing the body with live enzymes

You should commit to stop poisoning your cells with bad foods such as synthetics and indigestible foods. Replace this foods with natural, organic, whole foods. Natural foods, mostly raw foods contain live enzymes. Live enzymes are not found in processed foods. The enzymes act as catalysts for all human body functions. All humans have the capacity to produce an efficient load of enzymes, from birth. However, we have adapted to consuming processed foods which only use up our body enzymes without replacing them. Over time, we use up all our enzymes. We take the loss of enzymes as a slowdown of metabolic processes in the body systems. It is obvious that the body will slow down when it lacks enzymes which it uses in its functions. When you feed the body with live enzymes, your metabolism increases. You should consume a large amount of raw foods such as fruits and vegetables. They are enzyme rich and serve to improve the functioning of your body, especially the digestive system. Live enzymes are those that have not been exposed to heat or high temperatures. That is why it is best to eat raw foods to gain more live enzymes. A great amount of enzymes in the body serves to increase the amount of fuel in your body and give it potential for maximum production. Live enzymes also help in boosting and improving your energy levels. You will look and feel more vibrant. Live enzymes are good for the health of our bodies and general well-being. For those looking for a youthful look, live enzymes will do the trick. Live enzymes do all the dirty work of scrubbing out all the toxic dirt from your system. You need a plan of how you are going to incorporate the diets in your meals. Remember they are found in raw foods therefore salads would be a good start by having a variety of veggies and fruits in your salads. Instead of making smoothies or fruit juices, eat your fruits raw, mostly as snacks. A good routine that I have found working for me is eating fresh fruits only for breakfast at least thrice in a week. For lunch, have a substantial amount of vegetables for your salads. Some people prefer eating only uncooked plant foods for all meals but I would advise mixing your diet with cooked foods as well. You can divide your day into two parts. This way, you will have a wide range of options to choose between cooked foods and raw foods. You can have raw foods throughout the day for breakfast, brunch, lunch and snack hours. You can then have a cooked meal for dinner. You can also choose to combine raw and cooked foods for great digestion. The major advantage of eating raw foods before dinner is avoiding the fatigue caused by eating cooked foods during the day. A live enzyme based meal will ensure you eat light frequent meals throughout the day thus easing digestion and reducing fatigue. Lighter meals also increase your energy during busy working hours. You should eat heavy cooked meals at the end of the day. That is when the working hours are over and the energy is no longer required. However, the best approach in all this is trying out for yourself. Trying out the advice yourself will help you find out what works for you and what doesn't. It may be difficult for most people to adopt a raw dinner, since it is something they are not used to. You can try it for a few days a week to see how it goes for you.

Day to day detoxing

The body is exposed to harmful environmental toxins daily. The toxins are found in the air, water, food and different products that we use daily. The best detox program is a daily regime. We will provide you with simple and easy steps to help your daily detox routine. Your first reaction at realizing how much toxins your body can accumulate in a day, may be disgust and shock. These are understandable reactions. However, they should not be the reaction we focus or dwell on. They are not going to help our bodies get rid of the toxins that have built up. The built-in detox system is designed to remove many types of toxins found in the body. However, when overloaded, they cannot function efficiently. The results can be very dangerous and even fatal. The best way to ensure your body system is having an ongoing detox program. You can ensure proper functioning of your body's elimination system by utilizing simple daily steps. The body systems are empowered to carry out the functions they are meant to do. The immune system in the body is strengthened. There repair systems function more efficiently. Overall, your health, vitality and resilience is improved. This is even in the event of unpredictable challenges. The daily detox program doesn't require extreme dieting or unrealistic cleansing routines. It is a gradual process with sustainable results. It becomes a way of life. Below is a guide that will support the main elimination systems of the body which are; kidneys, intestines, skin, liver, lymphatic system, bowels and lungs. There is additional information on the causes of toxins accumulation. There are also signals sent out by the organs to display the increase in toxins levels which may affect their functions.

After the detox

As you finish the detox, you may realize that your tastes in food have changed. You may find yourself craving veggies, fruits and other foods you might not have desired before the detox. Your digestive system is relaxed during the detox period. Therefore you shouldn't consume hard to digest foods immediately after the detox. For example, do not consume French fries, pizza or other fast foods just a day after detoxing. You may want to reintroduce cooked veggies in your diet, gradually. Vegetable soups and broths are also great for the after detox period. Next, you can introduce whole grains, oils, dairy and meat in your regular diet, however, ensure the amounts of these foods are moderated. After detox, the appetite and food tastes for most people change. You should train yourself to adopt a vegetarian diet for long or as a lifestyle change. Doing so will help you enjoy the full benefits of the detox. After the detox program, you should continue practicing most of the healthy habits that you have learnt. After the detox, you can practice a maintenance version where you continue with a gentle detox. You can also end the detox diet and reintroduce foods in your regular diet. The best part of the program is to identify foods which you are sensitive, intolerant or allergic to. Do not reintroduce eliminated foods all at once. Introduce the foods one at a time over several days at intervals. For example, you can have wheat products twice a day in the first few days. Later, you can reintroduce, glutens and dairy. If you reintroduce all foods at once, you cannot know which foods are problematic.

Functions of the kidneys

- They control water, acid and mineral levels
- They regulate blood pressure
- Delivering oxygen to body cells
- They relay toxic signals through symptoms such as; dark urine and infrequent urination

There are factors which can lead to stressed functioning of the liver. They include;

- Dehydration
- High cholesterol intake

- Consumption of refined sugars
- Intake of low fiber content
- Consumption of high sodium amounts in food

Kidneys need a lot of water for proper functioning. Dietary needs may vary between individuals. However, the recommended amount is 80 to 120 ounces of water daily. You can also consume other healthy drinks such as herbal tea and fruit juices. Avoid going back to old bad habits. Do not consume caffeine or alcohol since they will leach water from the body, leaving insufficient amount for elimination processes. You should seek to reduce stress from the kidneys so that they can function properly. You can do this by practicing healthy habits which help in reducing blood pressure. They include; getting exercise daily and restricting sodium intake. This can be essential for people who experience increase in blood pressure when they consume high sodium content. LDL cholesterol should not be in high levels. This is because high levels of these can affect the functions of the kidney. You should increase intake of healthy foods. These foods include; walnuts, almonds and salmon. Brightly colored fruits and vegetables are good for the kidney. They help in reducing inflammation. You should reduce or completely eliminate consumption of unhealthy fats. Examples of fat sources are bacon and sausages. There are premade baked pastries which contain both trans-fats and saturated fats.

Functions of the liver

The liver removes a variety of toxins from blood. Other functions are as follows;
- Regulating sugar levels in blood
- Storing essential nutrients
- Disposes old red blood cells

The following are signs that the liver may be in a toxic state;
- Bloating

- Nausea
- Indigestion
- Eye whites turn yellow
- Yellow or white hue on the tongue

Factors that can cause the symptoms above are;

- Excessive consumption of alcohol
- Saturated fats

You should add lemons and limes in your water. On the other hand, refined sugar, flour, meat and dairy products are acidic. Therefore, consuming excessive amounts of acidifying foods causes the liver to develop fatty deposits and it cannot carry out its functions effectively. Alcohol, caffeine and sugar intake should be limited. Caffeine has stimulating effects which causes reactions in the body that can stress the liver. The reactions can also affect metabolic processes. White foods are not good for the liver since they increase blood sugar. They include; white bread, white rice and white flour. You should instead consume foods that scrub the liver. Celery, beets, asparagus and artichokes are also good for the liver.

Functions of the guts and entrails

Signs that the bowels and intestines may be in a toxic state are;

- Constipating
- Bad breath
- Bloating
- Diarrhea
- Skin breakouts

The following factors contribute to build up of toxins;

- A diet with low fiber content
- Consuming excessive amounts of processed foods
- Foods with high saturated fat content
- Pesticide residues in food
- Food allergies

Below are recommendations to ensure proper functioning of the bowels and intestines.

- Avoid foods which you may experience sensitivity to. They include; eggs, gluten, soy and dairy
- Eat fiber rich foods such as; figs, pears, black beans and berries
- Eat slowly and in manageable amounts. When you consume a lot of fiber, the body finds it difficult to process. Chew your foods till it becomes liquid before swallowing. That will make work easier for your digestive juices. A digestive enzyme supplement is also good for the process. You can take probiotics which contain a bacteria that makes digestive processes progress easily. Kefir and plain yoghurt also provide good bacteria. Constipation can be a symptom and cause of toxin buildup in the digestive system. Suffering chronic

constipation means the toxins in the body can be reabsorbed instead of being eliminated. To avoid constipation, drink more water, eat more fruits and vegetables. Yoga is also a good exercise to avoid constipation.

Roles of lungs

- filtering blood clots formed in the veins

Signs of toxicity in the lungs are;

- running nose
- clogged sinuses
- difficulty in breathing
- frequent sneezing and coughing

The following factors contribute to toxicity in the lungs

- cigarette smoke
- organophosphate fertilizers
- mold
- recycled air indoors

- dioxins
- traffic fumes
- recreational and medication drugs
- paint fumes
- exhaust fumes
- barbecue meat

Recommendations for avoiding toxicity in the lungs

- Quit smoking
- Reduce your intake of dairy
- Add ginger to your diet. You can add it to tea or foods as you cook
- There is a remedy proven effective for unblocking clogged sinuses. The water will clear the clogged nasal passages and come out through the other nostril.
- Read labels on detergents and other cleaning products. Follow the guidelines provided and ensure you work in a well-ventilated area. You can also opt to make cleaning products by

yourself. Use nontoxic ingredients when you do so.

- Eliminate household mold or mildew.
- Exercise daily. Ensure the exercises you choose makes your heart beat and make you breathe heavily. This will help in removing toxins from the lung tissues.

Functions of the Lymphatic system

The lymphatic system is made up of organs which prevent infection by clearing out waste and foreign materials from the body.

The following symptoms are an indication of toxicity in the lymphatic system;

- Exhaustion
- Puffy eyes
- Swollen nodes

Below are factors which may lead to the symptoms above;

- Unbalanced diet without enough fruits and vegetables
- Pesticide residues in the foods you eat

Recommendations

- Lymphatic massage: certified practitioners carry out this treatment to stimulate movement of lymphatic fluid. The treatment involves use light and brisk touches.
- Consume foods which boost your immunity. The foods include; carrots, red peppers and veggies
- Use cayenne pepper and horseradish in food flavoring. The spices enhance the circulation of lymphatic fluids
- Avoid using aluminum based deodorants. They block the system through which toxins are eliminated. Sweat is one ways through which toxins are eliminated and therefore you should allow your body to sweat
- Saunas and steam baths are a great way to stimulate sweating. They

enhance the process of lymph fluids circulation

Functions of the skin

The skin is the largest body organ. Its functions include;

- Blocking the external environment from internal body organs
- Regulating body temperature
- Moderating blood flow
- Excreting toxins

The signs below indicate that the skin is exposed to toxicity

- Rashes
- Acne
- Clogging of skin pores
- Skin flakes

The factors below contribute to the toxicity

- Inflammatory diet
- Using body care products which irritate the skin

- Using laundry products which may contain corrosive elements that affect the skin
- Pesticide residues on clothes
- Buildup of dead skin
- Overloading of body organs which leads to buildup of toxins

Make sure you read the ingredient labels on products, especially those with chemicals that come into contact with your skin. Avoid antiperspirants which contain aluminum since they prevent the skin from eliminating toxins through waste. There are beauty products which claim to be natural and organic. That is just a fad to market the product since there aren't any products which are processed and remain natural. For household cleaning products, avoid those with fragrances and dyes. Use products which don't contain fragrance and don't irritate the skin. Use bath scrubs to remove dead skin from the body and unclogging blocked pores. Equally the methods have a detoxing effect. Vigorous exercising helps your body detox since it will stimulate sweating. Saunas also helps unclog skin pores. Wear clothes made of cotton, hemp or line. They are kinder to the skin and more absorbent and breathable. Ensure the materials are organic to avoid pesticide residues which may be absorbed in the skin. Take healthy steps daily to keep away toxins from your body. When you do this, you will reap many health benefits. You feel energized and healthier when your natural detox benefits begin to kick in. your skin becomes clearer and metabolism increases. Small health problems disappear when you stick to a healthy diet. Detoxification is a major aspect in preventive medicine. It is safe, affordable and an easy solution to your health problems. Your body system functions better when you detox.

Detox Strategies

Detox strategies are all over the internet with every 'detox expert' having their own opinion. Most detox strategies are controversial, and have been dismissed to be just fads. So, do they actually work? Here is some advice from detox professional experts;

- Epsom salts and baking soda baths. Hot Epsom salt baths have been recommended as a detox strategy by medical practitioners. Some of the renowned doctors who have sworn by this strategy are Mark Hyman and Beverly Yates. The baths have a gentle and effective detox effect. They cleanse the body system. The effectiveness of the baths is attributed to their magnesium content. The function of the skin here in letting out toxins gives the kidneys a breather from performing this function. You can add baking soda to your Epsom salt baths. It helps in preventing dry skin.

- Detox footbaths. It is always a good feeling to soak your feet in warm water. Ionic footbaths have been known to have the effect of removing toxins through the feet. However, there is no scientific evidence to support this. When you soak your feet water and the water turns to a brown color, some claim that the color is caused by the toxins released from the feet. Attributing the brown color to dirt removed from the feet is more logical. Some have claimed the same effect is caused by the corrosive effect of ionic charge to the salts in the water. Detox foot pads are very essential in this process. They are held over steam and display dark stains.

- Master cleanse. It was founded in 1941 by Stanley Burroughs. Stanley advocated for consumption of raw foods. The Master cleanse involves fasting for ten days. During the fast, your consumption is limited to water containing lemon juice, cayenne pepper and maple syrup. Even today, the master cleanse is still recommended by doctors. One of the medical practitioners who has advocated for the master cleanse is Elson M. Haas He refers to master cleanse as a "spring cleanse". The master cleanse helps relieve congestion which may be caused by overindulging in processed foods. However, he supervises his detox clients carefully throughout the fast. If anyone is in poor health or is a first timer in fasting, they should seek medical guidance. The master cleanse is not recommended for those trying to lose weight. If you have weight issues such as obesity, you are advised to stick to long-term diet changes to avoid unhealthy programs which may worsen your condition.

- Colon cleanse. There are others who simply prefer having measured ingredients and dosage instructions. Majority of colon cleanse kits have a combination. They also contain sages.

- Colonic. These are proficient emetics. The process involves a health professional. The professional advises on how to use a combination of water and herbs for cleansing the colon. Colonics have been proven to remove waste and toxins from the body system. However, they are unnecessary and pose a risk to some groups of people for example those with chronic health issues. Colonics can disrupt the pressure of fluids in the colon. They can also cause imbalance of bacteria in the intestines and encourage unhealthy behaviors among participants.

Comparison between food and fasting

There is a difference between food based cleansing and fasting. When you fast or complete a juice cleanse, it means you are not consuming any solid foods and fiber. Your body is entirely relying on sugars for energy. The fasts ensure no energy is used by your digestive system, since no digestive processes take place. All the energy consumed is distributed to the rest of your body. The most common example of such fasts is the juice fast which mostly lasts from between three to ten days. Most fast programs require use of laxatives. They act as replacements for fiber and whole foods which are normally required by the body to eliminate wastes. Laxatives include; herbal teas and stimulants. The laxatives enhance the elimination of wastes and toxins in the body. However, fasting and laxatives are not recommended as healthy ways of fasting. Fiber is very essential in the detoxing process. During detoxification, the body releases wastes and toxins which buildup in the digestive tract. Whole foods such as fruit and vegetables contain natural fibers. Fiber absorbs toxins and waste in the body and removes them safely and easily from the body. Fibers also keep you feeling full by reducing the rate at which glucose is absorbed from food. Therefore when we don't consume fiber during a detox, it becomes difficult for the body to remove toxins. Fruits and vegetables in the juices we consume during fasts contain vitamins and antioxidants. However, the fiber element has been removed from the juices leaving just sugar and water. Fiber and protein are required to slow down digestion. When they lack in a diet, the blood sugar levels in the body rises. The rise causes insulin levels in the body to become unstable. The body requires fibers and proteins to maintain stability of blood sugar levels. The body is designed to function on whole foods. Most of the information available about metabolic damage is conflicting. Fasting may not have long-term effects on the metabolism. However, there are obvious disadvantages of fasting. The main disadvantage is the constant hunger pangs. If you still want to have a juice fast, you have two options. You can make your own cleanse juice or order pre-made juice. Both options can be pricey and not affordable to everyone, especially purchasing. Luxury juice cleanses ordered can set you back up to $100 a day. The costs accrue to such high amounts due to shipping costs. To imagine paying that much for plastic bottles containing mostly water across the country. The cost is expensive and the process is also bad for the environment since it leaves a large carbon footprint through transportation and packaging. If you are set on doing a juice fast, the best approach is easing in and out of it. Ensure you continue with the fast routine for a few more days before and after the fast, so as to transition smoothly. There are times which aren't conducive for one to fast, so as to avoid serious health consequences. Below are times you should avoid fasting;

- When pregnant
- When nursing (postnatal care)
- When you are recovering from ailments or injuries
- If you suffer from malnutrition
- If you have type 1 diabetes
- Heart diseases such as heart failure
- Kidney diseases
- Ulcers
- If you suffer mental illnesses such as anxiety and depression
- If you suffer eating disorders or are over ten pounds underweight
- If you are under regular medication, including antidepressants
- If you take birth control pills

If you are diabetic or constantly experience migraines, consult a medical professional before fasting.

Chapter 4:

Management of all the symptoms of detox

If You are probably worried about the symptoms of detx and you are wondering how you can get out of the situation don't worry. There are some testimonials from people who got out of such symptoms like kaeng raeng a customer who had the symptoms and didn't give up on herself. She said that her symptoms went for a day and included, cold chills at night, headaches, feeling nauseous and withdrawn but she realized these signs are similar to those of withdrawal, they were from salt fat and sugars as well as caffeine.

She realized her body was addicted to eating unhealthy foodstuffs. Th detox cleansed her body and made her get more insights on the lifestyle and healthy living practices. Her life improved and changed in a huge way after detoxing and making better food choices. The amount or levels of energy in the body is released after detoxing hence these symptoms are expected. The products of detoxing will have an effect on the body after the first twenty four hours. That's among the expected things to happen.

Let's learn more about detox symptoms and why they happen.

When you get symptoms after detoxing it means that the program worked for you!! There is no need to worry after getting these signs because it is usually an indication that your body is responding positively to the program. The impurities and toxins in the body once cleansed its normal for the body to respond and react hence the symptoms are expected to show. The bloodstream and the other skin and body systems are expected to react in one way or another after you detox. The discomfort that comes after detoxing is therefore normal hence you do not need to worry. The reactions vary hence you can't compare your symptoms with someone else's symptoms. The diet you choose and the following food choices will have a huge impact on your body too hence the reactions will depend on what you eat too.

If you notice some body reaction after following a certain diet its advisable to change the diet and try another type of diet. If its dairy products like meat, milk, cheese or sugars you can substitute that part of your diet with something else. The withdrawal symptoms however, cannot be avoided and do not necessarily mean that when you abstain from these types of foods you will feel any better. It just helps changing the diet. The healing crisis after detox or the herxheimer reaction as many call it is normal and the symptoms associated with it are called the detox symptoms. Do not let your response to the detox program get inside your head and get you worried. It's completely normal!!

Just like the testimony of Kaeng Raeng,the program helps cleanse your system and if you have been trying using some laxatives with your program, the negative side effects are expected.

What to expect after your detox program is over.

Just like after consuming something new, the side effects normally show, the detox program shows side effects and these are shown as symptoms after cleansing.

You can learn from customer experiences and experiences after trying the program that the symptoms will obviously show after finishing your program. The common issue is usually consumption of water and this helps as well as consumption of smoothies after finishing the program. The body adapts after the program as it cleanses the bowels and skin as well a other systems of the body. The toxins from each part of the body and all the systems is eliminated through the program. You should expect to see your body reacting in one way or another and the symptoms are expected.

Make sure that you drink the required glasses of water after detoxing and you will feel a less effect of the cleansing process. The other thing that you should get is enough rest and sleep. The main area of emphasis is staying hydrated and also resting enough. The energy used in the detox process will call for enough rest because the energy required in the process is a lot of energy.

Here are herbs and Supplements you can take to enhance your cleansing process

It is proven that taking some supplements with your detox program can aid in your cleansing process. The supplements can be incorporated in a diet too and they work best in enhancing how te detox program works.

Enhance your detox process and get the most out of it in these ways;

Among the best ways of enhancing your cleansing process, exercising on routine basis can help in releasing toxins as it lets out the sweat and improves general blood circulation.

- Through aerobics, the heart and blood circulation is enhanced hence the detox process gets better and works faster.

- The other main thing is staying hydrated and drinking enough water in a day as you listen to the way your body responds. The toxins can be released faster if you sweat more hence staying hydrated and exercising enhances your detox process.

- Go for a massage often when you are detoxing as the skin helps in elimination of toxins. When you get a massage your body can easily release toxins too. All these are ways of attaining your cleansing goals faster and easily.

Chapter 5:

How to maximize the potential benefits of a natural detox

The most highly recommended way of enhancing your detox experience is by increasing blood circulation and sweat. The toxins must be eliminated from the body eventually. The best, easiest and quickest way to do so is by ensuring your heart is pumping. Engage in exercises that get you sweating. Such exercises include aerobics and hot yoga. The exercises speed up the process of detoxification. Exercise caution while exercising to prevent any risk of injury or over-exerting your body. When you exercise, you will sweat and lose water in the body. Keep hydrated by drinking plenty of water. Dehydration and excessive sweating can lead to electrolyte loss. When you fast, aerobic exercise is not recommended. Saunas are a great way of enhancing the detox process. A sauna will cause you to sweat, thus stimulating release of toxins quickly through the skin. Body massages also help in quickly moving toxins through the body. Therefore, you will not only be treating yourself, but helping your body eliminate toxins in the process. For body massage, it is best to involve a professional massage therapist. They are well versed in detox procedures and treatments. They can offer massages tailored to your detox needs. Such massages include; massaging the kidneys and increase of blood flow in the lower body.

Exercise

A detox doesn't mean you have to stop all exercise routines. However, you should avoid strenuous exercises. Stick to gentle exercises such as power walks. Power walks include long and quick paced steps where you walk for around fifteen minutes in a day. Yoga and tai chi are also great exercises during a detox. Spend time outdoors to get some fresh air and sunshine. It will feel good on your skin, will be beneficial for your body and will uplift your moods. However, do not get too cold or get too much sun. Treat your body with gentleness. In turn, the body devotes most of its resources to heal and cleanse itself. Take time to carefully examine the toxic load in your body. Find ways of reducing exposure elements that cause toxicity. A detox plan requires commitment and willingness. If you are devoted to the course, you will enjoy the benefits because it works. Strictly follow a detox plan even for just a week and you will notice the beneficial impact it will have on your body and overall well-being. A detox helps in increasing your energy levels and leaving you with bright feelings. It helps you gain clarity of the mind.

A healthy detox is not about denying yourself or self-indulgence. You will learn this from your personal detox experience. It is also not about taking pills or wrapping yourself up in seaweed. A good detox is about creating a healthy and sustainable lifestyle.

Paraben, Phthalate. What are they?

You may be familiar with the phrases 'paraben free and cruelty free' in skin care products. But do you really know what it means? Such products include; make-up, body lotions, hair shampoos and toothpaste. Parabens are artificial lab-made chemicals. They are extremely cheap, which is why most manufacturing companies prefer to use them. It is an economical gain for them, at the expense of the consumer's health. They are used in fighting bacteria and fungus therefore they are also common in some anti-bacterial and anti-fungal creams. They are also used in preservatives, and can preserve skin care products such as lotions for up to 50 years. According to dermatology research, absorption of parabens by the skin and eventually into the body is very dangerous for your health. Studies have been conducted by the Environmental Working Group which had some concerning results. They showed that parabens can lead to the following diseases;

- Cancers such as breast cancer
- Immuno-toxicity
- Skin irritation
- Endocrine disruption
- Reproductive issues such as infertility
- Toxicity to the neural system

In 2004, a study was conducted among 20 women who had breast cancer. Out of the 20 participants, traces of parabens were found in the tumors of 19 participants. The link between parabens and cancer cannot be taken lightly. The study detected intact parabens which were unchanged by metabolic processes in the body.

It is worrying to note that they are also used in pharmaceutical industry and baby care products, considering their harmful effects. They are absorbed through the skin into the body and have been linked to health issues such as;

- Birth defects
- Asthma
- Obesity
- Infertility
- Hormonal imbalance
- Birth defects
- Asthma

They also affect neurodevelopment in newborns. The products do not use artificial chemicals and preservatives in manufacturing. They use gentle ingredients which are safe for humans to use every day on their skin. Cruelty free ensures animals are not hurt at the expense of human beings. Protecting animals from tests and human research is a great conservation and preservation effort of the natural environment. It is important to have concern over animals' health, safety and wellbeing. Therefore, we should use products that are free from parabens, phthalates and cruelty free. Also, have a short-time detox.

The skin secret, which is exfoliation

Exfoliation helps in having a healthy detox. When shopping for skin care products, get a natural based ingredients exfoliator. Another good way of taking care of your skin is through dry brushing. The process stimulates the lymphatic system and aids it in moving of toxins through the body and eventually eliminating the toxins. Dry brushing clears the excess dead skin, causing the pores to open up. When the pores are open, they excrete toxins from the body efficiently. Here is a great guide for skin brushing;

- Dry brush before showering. Begin with light pressure
- Avoid synthetic and nylon material brushes since they can irritate the skin
- Begin the process at the soles of your feet
- Afterwards, start with the hands, arms and towards your heart
- Brush the back
- Brush the abdomen, chest and neck. Do not brush the face because its skin is more sensitive.
- The brushing process should take between three to five minutes.
- After brushing, take a shower to remove the dead skin
- Ensure you don't share your dry brush and wash it every once in a while
- After showering, apply a natural oil to the skin

Remember to avoid skin products which have toxic chemicals since they will set you back in your detox journey. There are other ways to speed up the process of detoxification. However, they are not recommended to everyone since they are forceful. One such procedure is colon hydrotherapy. It involves sending water to the colon and draining it out with a tube. The procedure is very risky and dangerous and would not be recommended for anyone with pre-existing medical conditions. The biggest risk is damaging the colon, which is most likely irreversible. The colon may become dependent on the procedure for it to function. The muscles of the colon may fail to stimulate on their own therefore paralyzing colon function. Therefore wastes in the colon may get stuck. Salt water goes through the body without being absorbed. It flushes out nearly everything in the colon. However, this procedure is unpredictable and is therefore not recommended due to the health risks it poses.

Top detoxing tips

1. **Avoiding white food stuffs**. They include refined sugar and flour. They negatively affect your energy levels. They overload the major organs in the body especially the kidneys and liver. You should only consume foods which boost your detox process. Such foods include; fruits, vegetables, whole grains, nuts and seeds. Try to eat natural organic foods as much as possible.

2. **Avoid bad fats**. They include; saturated fats and trans-fats. Bad fats affect the functioning of body systems. The liver is the most affected. It becomes slower in its functioning when it is exposed to unhealthy fats.

3. **Stay Hydrated**. You should consume plenty of water at all times, daily. Water is very essential in the detox process. It helps in flushing out

wastes. Adding lime or lemon to your drinking water helps in boosting your detox. Limes and lemons contain alkaline elements that support detoxification. Avoid soft drinks, even diet soda. Also be mindful of drinks which contain high levels of caffeine or stimulants.

4. **Check your household products**. Most household products such as paint, air fresheners and sealants contain VOCs. VOCs are volatile organic compounds. The compounds cause headaches, nausea, liver and kidney damage. Purchase VOC free products.

5. **Be very selective on by oils – the lotions** we use contain dangerous chemicals. Be aware of the toxic ingredients that can harm your skin. Read the ingredients lists to know what a product contains. Do not always fall for the 'natural' and

'organic' marketing gimmicks on most skin care products.

6. **Release stress**. Stress causes toxicity in the body. It affects our hormone reactions causing hormonal imbalance and release of hormones which cause feelings such as sadness. Such hormones can lead to mental health issues such as depression and anxiety. Stress affects the functioning of body systems by overloading them with toxic byproducts. Find out and engage yourself in activities which help you in relaxing. Examples of such activities are; yoga, meditation, nature walks and body massage. Carry out the activities often and consistently. Incorporate them in your daily routines and schedules. Doing this will help you get rid of unhealthy stress and help your body retain the benefits of a detox.

Liver Detox

The liver is found on the right side of the abdomen. It is one of the major organs in the body system. Some of these functions make it possible to lose and manage weight healthily. The liver carries out many metabolic processes and other functions such as;

- Supporting the digestive system
- Controlling blood sugar
- Regulating storage of body fats
- Storing and mobilizing energy
- It produces the largest amount of proteins in the body
- It conducts the chemical breakdown of everything entering the body. The range is from healthy organic foods to poisonous chemicals in food additives. It also processes drinking water, wine, alcohol, diet supplements and medication.

The liver is tasked with differentiating between healthy nutrients which should be absorbed in the body It also has an important function of processing nutrients and fats. If your body is full of toxins, you will have more difficulty losing weight and maintaining your ideal weight. It is ironic that most of the low carb diets that people adopt only serve to worsen the situation. The low carb diets encourage us to consume a lot of meat. Note that most meat we eat has a lot of toxins. The diet also discourages consumption of fiber rich foods and water-dense fruits and vegetables. Lacking these in a diet slows down elimination. The low carb diets load our bodies with excessive amounts of proteins. The stomach is unable to produce enough acid to digest the proteins. The diets prevent proper digestion. They overload the liver and intestines with poisons which are produced internally. The poisons include; ammonia, cadaverine, indicant and histide. The liver produces bile, which is important in the detoxing process. Bile provides lubrication to the intestines and utilizes fiber to prevent constipation. The liver deposits the following toxins in bile;

- Industrial chemicals
- Heavy metals such as mercury and arsenic
- Drugs
- Excess sex hormones caused by birth control medication
- Pesticides

The toxins are absorbed by bile and eliminated from the body. One of the major functions of bile is helping the body to break down fats that we require for assimilation of fat soluble vitamins. Other functions of bile include; converting betacarotene into vitamin A and helping the body utilize calcium. However, bile can be overwhelmed in its functions by excessive toxins in the body. Therefore, liver detox is important in ensuring it produces better and more efficient bile which will help the body in breaking down fats and eliminating toxins. It also provides more nutrients in the body which give energy. When the body has enough energy, the digestive and immune systems are relieved of their strain. Elimination of toxins improves and the colon is not strained. It also cleans the entire body system. The program is tested and proven to be highly effective and healthy. It also comprises of a weight loss program that helps you lose weight in a simple, safe and effective way. You are able to clear out the toxins in your body, thus improving your health and vitality. There is a book known as 'Fast Track Detox Diet' which has more details about this program. The diet will enhance a healthy lifestyle. It will put your mind at ease to know that it has been clinically tested and proven to be safe and effective. There is one-day fast in the detox program, therefore it is safe and you won't have to starve while detoxing. The complete detox program requires you to prepare for seven days and ease into the program within three days. It is set up in such a way to ensure your body system is fully prepared for the single day juice fast whose main aim is detoxing your liver. The one day fast will help in extending and compounding your healthy gains. The detox program has the following benefits;

- Improving liver and colon state and functioning
- Cleansing body tissues
- Getting rid of bloating
- Improving your energy levels
- Help you lose weight
- It is safe and gentle
- Improves your health and vitality

The program is better than the popular water fasting. It is easy and can be practiced anytime you feel a drop in your energy levels. It is highly recommended that you practice the program quarterly, at least once every three months. The best times are around fall and spring. However, do not limit yourself. Practice the program whenever you feel sluggish and overloaded with toxins. An additional benefit is how easy it is to incorporate the program into your everyday routine. For a whole week, you consume the foods that your liver needs to function effectively. The foods will work great not just on your liver but your body system in general. Also consume the foods that are colon friendly. Your colon will eliminate wastes and toxins from the body better. Afterwards, set aside a day for a juice fast. The juice fast will help you eliminate impurities and wastes that have accumulated in your body system. Finally, the three day sequel. It included more support for the liver and colon. It also includes consuming natural foods full of probiotics. You will consume fermented foods which work with healthy bacteria in synthesizing vitamins and boosting immunity in the body system. Many participants of the program reported significant and sustainable weight loss. However, we cannot overlook the long-term benefits, which are energy boost and better health. Whether your focus is on losing weight or eliminating toxins from your body, the fast track detox will work great for you. You will be amazed with the results your body can accomplish with just a little help.

CHAPTER 6:

Strategies of consuming a natural diet

How you can eat quick exit foods in some quick exit combination

After stopping cell poisoning, you need to learn about the secrets of eating foods that can enable you lose weight and the best way of eliminating body waste. The digestive system is the core of your secret because it controls how food moves in your body. When food moves fast in your digestive system it means that it will be eliminated fast too. That's the only way to reduce body waste accumulation. To attain this goal, you need to eat easily digestible foods and make sure you eat them in quickly exit combination for efficient results. This strategy in short lies on the theory that when food is digested faster, it reduces the chances of leaving waste matter. Keep in mind that if you are eating foodstuffs that take longer periods to get digested he body uses more energy and requires more resources to break down the food. This aids in a faster way of cleansing your body from all sorts of toxins. If you want to attain your weight loss goals, this is what you need. The combination of quick exit foods has been known to also help in reduction of digestive disorders like farting, constipation and irritable bowel syndrome among others. This combination helps you lose weight easily so to attain your body goals.

There are some foods you can eat with this combination to get positive results faster. Others take more time to digest like avocado. When you combine an avocado with certain foods you will notice differences in your digestive tract. The slower the digestion the slower the performance of the exit combination. This could lead to some effects on your digestive tract like arthritis, asthma and spleen issues as well as bacterial infections in the colon and the whole digestive tract. Constipation, acne can also be caused by issues with the digestive system. As you know, such stomach disorders drain your body energy hence you feel drained exhausted and overworked.

Learn more about the combination of quick -exit

First things first, there are generally four types of food categories which is flesh, starch, fresh fruits and dried fruits like nuts and seeds. Fruits and starch cannot be mixed in this food combination hence you need to carefully watch the combinations. It's advisable to mix the combinations with vegetables too for faster and best results. Ensure that the four combinations do not end up being in the stomach at the same time. Balance your intake of the four categories wisely. Remember that there is usually diversity in people's digestive tracts hence you should not compare your response with someone else's response to these foods.

If you want to know that a certain combination of these foods works best for you, just experiment on your body.

When you notice that you are still losing weight and your gastrointestinal tract works normally that is you aren't feeling any stomach discomfort then you can tell that the combination is working perfectly for you. Follow your specific rules and guidelines as you eat the food but keep in mind that self-discipline is key when you are serious about attaining specific body goals. For most individuals, they noticed that without following specific rules and being self-disciplined you don't get positive results soon. It takes a lot of commitment and sacrifice to get positive results. If you want to attain your cleansing and detox goals, you need to be serious about the way you carry out your routine practices.

Tips for the combination of quick exit

1. Know that there are generally some types of foodstuffs which you cannot mix in some meals. Like I have explained earlier when consuming some food rich in starch like avocado you need to be cautious. Dried fruits like nuts also need to be taken in moderate amounts to avoid too much effects on the digestive tract.

2. Note that avocados are an exception in this combination so be cautious when taking foods rich in starch.

3. Do not consume fruits when your stomach is empty. It's unhealthy so ensure that you will eat fruits after three hours from your previous meal intake.

4. Know that there are some foods that take up to thirty minutes to exit the stomach. Mostly try consuming fresh fruits to avoid this.

5. Bananas are among the best fresh fruits you can try consuming and they combine well with other types of fruits. Like avocadoes and nuts for instance.

6. Avoid eating fresh fruits for desserts after eating a meal because it may cause fermentation

7. Do not switch food groups until three or four hours have finished after eating a meal.

8. In case your appetite is good, eat more foodstuffs which are in the same food group.

9. Enjoy eating vegetables with all flesh dishes. Vegetables are usually among the best things to incorporate in your diet as it goes hand in hand with the food group you will choose.

10. Starch and several vegetables go hand in hand. Try that combination often to have a healthy lifestyle.

11. Combine dairy products with flesh. This also helps in making your life healthy and the digestive tract functions well.

12. Avoid placing nut butter on the grain breads.

13. Every time you are eating a raw meal ensure your recipe has several fresh fruits combined in the diet.

14. Combine corn as a common vegetable in your diet. It's something you can enjoy during the summer time.

15. In case you are planning to skip or miscombine the meal ensure its dinner.

16. Ensure the meal with starch have the foods with high levels like grains and so on.
17. Have distinct rules as you make good food choices.
18. Use chocolates as desserts for any food category. When you choose a food category use chocolate as desserts because it has less milk or sugars.
19. You can mix dairy products too with any food combination but make wise food group choices.

The combination of slow exit

When you mix diverse food categories some things are bound to happen. For instance after eating flesh foodstuffs your tummy will send pepsin which digests proteins as the principal enzyme to initiate digestion.

After eating starch foods your tummy sends the alkaline digestive enzymes to aid in digestion. When alkaline and acidic enzymes neutralize in the stomach fermentation occurs. If there are inhibitors to digestion, bacteria slows down digestion and may lead to sickness, constipation or diarrhea. When you have digestive issues your body may not be able to fight diseases due to energy loss and low immunity. In order to maintain organs and tissues upkeep you need to make good food choices.

When the circulation of blood is poor the detox process is also inhibited in one way or another. The process of food elimination slows down if you have issues in your food combination. But when you have the right combination of food you eat what you love and you get to enjoy the best combination of food. Natural foods rarely cause digestive tract disorders and the best way to know a combination of food has an effect on your digestive system is by figuring out how gassy you get after eating food. When you combine your foods well you can easily attain your body weight goals.

Learn about the neutral foodstuffs

When you want to attain your best combination of food the neutral foodstuffs works best with all food combinations except the fresh fruits. If you are wondering what the neutral foodstuffs entail here is a list:

- raw vegetables
- Chocolate
- Condiments like mustard and soy sauce
- olive oil,
- herbs
- spices
- other seasonings

- Almond milk
- hot chocolate made with nut milk
- honey
- pure maple syrup

The non-neutral food stuffs entail:

- Lemons
- tomatoes

Real-Life scenarios

Eating in restaurants

Don't worry about your cleansing lifestyle of detoxification because you love eating take out or just hotel food. The natural diet of detoxification can be followed even if you are a restaurants kind of person. Just order what you eat in your normal diet at home. Do not compromise your daily diet and inhibit your body goals achievement. If you find it hard sticking to a food plan then avoid eating in hotels and eateries. Strive hard to achieve your cleansing and body goals.

Here are some tips you can use for fast foods eateries.

When ordering take out try getting some garden salad that has cucumbers, red onions, carrots and grape tomatoes. Avoid cheese use sea salt instead for top dressing. Stay away from fried foods, instead try the boiled take outs. Try to stay away from carbonated drinks like sodas and you should try eating natural nuts often. Try drinking herbal tea or naturally sweetened foods and drinks. Try taking lemon water as often as possible to promote your general lifestyle. Buy lemonade often!!

What to do when dining at family gatherings or private dinners and social events

I know you wonder from time to time how you can behave as someone's guest.

Telling your host that you are detoxing and you are following a certain diet may be weird. You may not want to sound rude but remember you are on a detox plan and the main thing to do is adhere to your food plan despite the fact that you are at a friend's house. Choose wisely what to eat at a friend's house if there is a salad go for it. Fresh vegetables and a delicious salad would be perfect if you are at a friend's house for dinner.

That way you can easily avoid awkward moments and be respectful at the same time without compromising your food plan. For formality just tell the friends that you are on a diet and then act freely as you enjoy your meal together. The same case applies if you are on a social event. If you are at a family gathering be open and feel free to tell your family members that you are on a diet. The other thing to keep in mind is that in all the events you should consume a lot of fruits and vegetables. Just make the right food choices despite the location or situation, never compromise your detox food plan. It's your duty to practice the best self-control and obedience when you are on a diet.

Buffets and barbeque gatherings

You may have wondered how to act when you have been invited for a barbeque or a formal and casual meals. Don't worry about the response to give to your friends during such occasions. Just be genuine and begin by telling them that you are on a diet. That way there will be no awkward moments between you or your friends.

When picking what to put in your plate start with natural salads. Add some raw corn to your diet. Choose meat wisely and avoid consuming a fruit after you have finished your meal. Carry a bar of chocolate in your bag to act as the dessert when you are done eating your meal.

Holiday seasons food plan strategies

You know how tempting holiday seasons can get, that because of the various vacations and events involved. Statistically many people gain up to ten pounds during holidays because people get relaxed and spend a lot of time lazing around. But what can we say and that's what makes holidays and vacations fun moments. However if you are serious about your cleansing process there are several things that you should avoid for your own safety. Do not let these fun moments distract you or compromise your detox process if it is snacks, just watch what you eat and stay cautious. Try your way to stick to your food plan and avoid all the complications that come with being disobedient and lacking perseverance.

Avoid alcohol consumption during your holiday or vacation. Split you vacation festivities and have control over what you eat.

Choose your starches wisely and eat natural foods, I insist eat natural vegetables. Try eating fruits for breakfast during your vacation. Enjoy your holiday meal but do not eat under stress influence.

Natural detox diet on a limited budget

For beginners in detoxing, a natural diet may seem a bit costly as compared to your regular diet. It may be actually costly, since you will have to replace the foods you normally consume. However, the high costs are just experienced in the beginning. That is because you will need to buy new items in the kitchen. After you make the initial purchases, maintaining the flow will be less expensive. When I used to shop in traditional supermarkets, I would spend averagely $750 per month on groceries alone. At the time, my roommate and I would eat between four and six meals out weekly. Currently, I spend the same amount of money on grocery shopping. However, I now prepare most of the meals in the house to avoid buying cooked and packaged foods. I use very high quality natural ingredients therefore it's a good bargain for my money and health. I can tell there is a big difference between the home-made meals and purchased food. Packaged food is very expensive. It is ironic that the lowest income earners make the highest number of consumers of packaged foods. It may be due to the fact that most low income earners work menial jobs for example in industries, and don't have enough time to prepare their own food. They also cannot afford to buy fresh healthy cooked foods. Due to these factors, the society is suffering from an influx in cases of lifestyle diseases such as; obesity and diabetes. If you are on a tight budget, it is advised that you consume natural foods. After all, you cannot afford the expensive medical treatment for most lifestyle diet related diseases. When you eat healthy, you will be naturally beautiful. You won't require to spend a lot of money on makeup, clothes and other cosmetic treatments. However, there is an interesting comparison between store bought cosmetics and natural products. A jar of raw almond butter costs around $7. When you buy peanut butter in a store, it sets you back around $4. The raw almond butter is a healthier choice. It has raw enzymes, calcium and protein which can be absorbed in the body for a healthy boost. The peanut butter you buy in stores contains preservatives, high salts and sugars which cannot be processed by the body. You will eventually realize that cheap is expensive. It is better to spend a larger amount of money on natural products than products with salt, sugar and preservatives. Natural products will save you a trip to the hospital with dietary diseases and other lifestyle diseases. If you are on a budget, you should eat economically. There are whole grains such as millet and brown rice which are healthy, cheap and filling. Sweet potatoes and sprout grain bread are also great options. Purchase your fresh fruits, vegetables, grains and raw nuts at inexpensive grocers. If you can afford to, it is cheaper to stock up in bulk on these products. Remember that treats are a bit pricier. However, we all deserve a little treat every once in a while. Research on the prices of products online and find the best offers. There is a healthy diet option tailored for every budget out there. Another way to go about this is assess the areas of your life where you may be spending money unwisely. A weekly visit to a spa and beauty salon is not a necessity. Impulse buying and expensive coffee dates should take a break. Cut out on expenses which are not necessities. Learn how to prioritize your health and well-being. You have only one life and one body that you cannot replace. Therefore, give it the best care. Below are a few foods and products that you can consume for your natural detox.

- Vegetable soup
- Brown rice
- Sweet potatoes
- Raw almonds
- Avocados
- Bananas
- Dates
- Raw walnuts
- Apples

How to maintain a natural detox diet in the office

For the time I have worked with business people in office settings, I know that this program can be implemented in an office. Below are guide steps on practicing the program in an office.

- Make double amounts of raw salad dressing and other foods that can be stored. Keep half of the foods at home and bring the other half to refrigerate in the office. This way, you can always enjoy foods you prepared yourself, right in the office

- Pack a bag of fresh fruits to take to the office daily. The best types are; bananas, grapes and other fruits which will not create a mess. Have a sharp knife and spoon in the office to cut up, slice and eat your fruits.

- Have some healthy treats such as nuts in a drawer. The snacks do not require refrigeration. However, eat them within two weeks.

- Plan for office meetings and parties. Common events in the office are; birthdays, engagements and baby showers. Always store healthy beverages such as herbal tea, to drink during such occasions. You are allowed some dark chocolate and a slice of cake, occasionally.

When you begin the program, it may be difficult at first to follow it in an office setting. Your colleagues may find it disturbing at first and even try to discourage or distract you from following the program. However, stay true to your course. Do not take a glazed doughnut just because someone says you should. On the other hand, do not beat yourself up when you occasionally indulge in sweet treats. Just be self-aware of your habits and keep focused on your goal.

Chapter 7:

Guidelines to sustain your detox

It is delicious, convenient, filling and easy to prepare. We have prepared you recipes of smoothies, salads and a whole lot more range of delicious foods and beverages to enjoy during your detox program. Most people use only water during a detox. Others prefer to mix with non-dairy milks, healthy juices and smoothies. It all depends on preference, since all options are great. Be careful of added refined sugars which contain unwanted calories. You can also use fruits and veggies in your smoothies. During a three day cleanse, ensure you eat lots of fruits and vegetables. An easy way of increasing your consumption of fruits and veggies is using them for your smoothies. It should be noted that a detox program is a chance for your body to rest from processing toxins and chemicals. It is advisable to use filtered water in your smoothies.

A weeks period prologue

Fasting can be hazardous if done wrongly. Let me explain why. Fasting leads to the release of toxins which were stored in fat cells. The toxins are transported to the bloodstream to be filtered and transported through the elimination organs of the body. The liver and colon should be prepared in advance to remove the toxins from the body. If this is not done, the toxins will relocate to other areas in the body. They can be absorbed by sensitive organs which can lead to feelings of; fatigue, anxiety and migraines. Below are six steps which when combined with your regular diet, can help in supporting the detox process. Follow them for seven days before you begin your juice fast.

1. Eat;

- Leafy vegetables and herbs; collards, kale, mustard greens and watercress
- Citrus fruits; limes, oranges and lemons. Do not eat grapefruit. It contains a compound known as naringen which can interfere with detox process in the liver
- Foods containing sulfur; eggs, garlic, daikon radish and eggs
- Liver healing foods; beets, artichoke, whey, asparagus and celery

2. A minimum of;
- Carrots
- Berries
- Pears
- Apples
- flax seeds

The foods in this category are good for the colon

3. Drink purified water.

4. Have a minimum of two portions of proteins daily. Examples of the best proteins to consume are; lean beef, turkey, fish, lamb and skinless chicken. For vegans and vegetarians, have a minimum of 2tbsp of blue-green algae daily.

2 tablespoons of olive or flaxseed oil daily.

5. Avoid the following, which can negatively affect a detox;

- Excessive consumption of dietary fats such as
- Soy foods
- Alcohol
- Artificial sweeteners
- Caffeine
- Refined carbohydrates
- Gluten

Tips for detox shopping

1. Make several copies of the foods and ingredients you need. Keep a list in your purse, car, kitchen and office drawers

2. If the nearest health food store is a couple of miles away, keep the wrappers of the foods you buy. Use the wrappers in asking around the local stores and market for the products. You can also decide to purchase in bulk, which is a cheaper option since you buy at wholesale price. If you purchase in bulk, the company can deliver directly to you.

3. Search for farming cooperatives. They offer a variety of fresh fruits and veggies at budget friendly prices

4. Don't just buy foods since it's a habit. You will end up buying the same produce too often and get bored with the routine. You will also be missing

out on what other products have to offer. Buy at least a new fruit and vegetable each week. Buying a new type of produce every now and then will help you try out new recipes.

5. Quit focusing on what you can't have and shift your attention to everything you can have

6. Clear your pantry of all the bad foods you want to eliminate from your diet. Replace these foods with healthy natural foods. If you have a family, leave them some of the foods you are eliminating. It wouldn't be fair to force them on your diet

7. Familiarize yourself with produce and bakery managers of local stores. Produce managers will help you find fresh produce. They can even order for you items you need that they don't stock or have run out of. Bakery managers will help you with healthy treats such as raw gourmet. Having

such options is a great lifesaver for a detox program.

8. Find a nearby health food store to stock up on the healthy foods you need. Such stores are spread out almost at every corner in streets especially in cities

9. Buy extra produce than what you think you need, especially for beginners. When you start trying out the recipes in the diets, you will find yourself going for extra helpings. Having extra ingredients and produce will be helpful. Remember you will be eating lots of fruit which will build your appetite. Ensure you have enough fresh fruits and vegetables to eat to satisfaction.

10. Learn to enjoy the shopping process. We lead very hectic lives, with daily ups and downs. However, do not take shopping for what you need as a tiring hassle. Allow yourself to enjoy foods

that you love and that excite you. You may find yourself in situations where you are forced to wait in queue for long so as to make a purchase. Just breathe and relax. Think of all the great things recipes you will prepare with the ingredients. Think of how tasty they will be and how they will help your body in detoxifying. Think of the physical benefits you will gain.

A Day Fluid Fast

Its main aim is removing impurities from the liver and other cellular tissues. It supports your overall health and boosts your energy. However, clinically proven research has shown that short term juice fasts which are supported by nutritional preparation are great boosters of good health. During a detox, the colon requires adequate amounts of fiber. A juice fast can help you maintain long-term weight loss and a range of other health benefits. A juice fast helps your digestive system take a break from the regular amount of work it is used to. That contributes to more energy being free which can be used to heal and regenerate body cells and organs. Your calorie intake will also be limited for a single day. However, this period is too short to cause significant changes to your metabolism or cause starvation. Every ingredient used in the juice is specifically tailored to keep away hunger and balance blood sugar. It also stimulates your metabolism, keeps you feeling great and gives you energy for the whole day. You may experience some symptoms during the juice fast day. Most symptoms are general, but some are specific to individuals since everyone is unique. Here is a basic guide to follow on the juice fast day;

1. Prepare the juice. What to note about the ingredients; the cranberry juice should be unsweetened, the spices

should be ground and the juices freshly squeezed.

The program should begin in the morning, as soon as you wake up. It doesn't have to start at a specific time. However, ensure you have taken eight glasses of juice by the end of the day. You should additionally take 72 ounces of water by the end of the day. In the morning and the end of the day, have a serving of colon care supplements. Below are a few options of colon supplements to choose from;

- Ground flaxseeds which should be mixed with water or juice
- Powdered psyllium husks

During the fast, you should only perform light exercises. Such exercises include; 15 minute walks and mellow yoga. Do not engage in strenuous exercises since you will not have enough energy for them and you may end up injuring yourself.

Detox program recipes

Daybreak packet

- 3 glasses of water
- ½ cup of pineapple juice
- ½ a banana
- ½ a cup of berries

Joy Packet

- A cup of ice
- ½ cup of lemon juice
- ½ cup strawberries

Carrot-Mango Smoothie

- ½ cup of carrot juice
- ½ cup of mango fruit diced into huge junks

Antioxidant juice

- ½ cup of mixed berries
- Ice (optional)

Tropical Juice

- 2 cups of water
- coconut H2O
- mango chunks

Green juice

- 3 cups of H2O
- A cup of finely chopped veggies
- diced banana
- ice

Blend the ingredients together

Kale salad

- Two bunches of kale
- One avocado (ripe)
- Lemon juice freshly squeezed from one lemon
- One clove of garlic
- 1 tsp sesame oil
- Grated carrot
- Red onion
- Pepper of your choice

Method

- Place avocado and garlic in a bowl. Add sesame oil and lemon juice
- Mix the combination with the kale for around four minutes. The kale should appear dark and feel tender

- Place in the refrigerator to chill. You need to prepare the salad before other dishes to give it enough time to chill before serving.

Rabbit salad

- Celery stalks
- Lemon juice (freshly squeezed)
- Organic humus
- Baby carrots
- Cucumber

Rainbow salad

The name speaks for itself. The salad is made by a combination of ingredients which have different colors.

- Blueberries
- Red cherry tomatoes
- Yellow bell pepper
- Orange butternut
- Green spinach
- Purple beetroot

All the ingredients should be whole. Add the seeds to boiling water and let them boil for ten minutes. Enjoy the tea after taking your meals. You can have it every day during your detox. Other teas which are great during detox are ginger and licorice tea

Vegetarian chili

The recipe serves ten. Ensure you use organic ingredients as much as possible.

- Soup pot
- Seven cups of water (unfiltered)
- 2 yams, large size
- 3 cloves of garlic, crushed
- minced orange zest
- white onion
- stewed tomatoes
- 2 tbsp. of chili powder
- ½ cup minced cilantro
- Salt and pepper

Method

- Bring water to boil
- Add the mixture to the soup and stir
- Add beans, orange zest, bay leaf and cilantro to soup

- Add salt and pepper
- Simmer chili for 12 minutes
- Remove from heat when the yams are tender
- Serve hot

Baked beans breakfast recipe

If you want baked beans, you can walk into any grocery and buy a tin of baked beans. But here is why you shouldn't. Packed baked beans have a high salt and sugar content. However, it won't take you a lot of time or effort to make your own healthy and delicious baked beans. The recipe below originates from England, and the results are savory.

Ingredients

- ½ cup of dried beans of your choice
- Salt
- 1 tsp paprika
- 1 tsp mustard
- Tomato paste
- 2 sprigs of spring onion

- Apple cider vinegar

Method

- Soak the beans overnight
- Drain the beans and cook under low heat for an hour
- When they are tender, drain the water
- Chop the onions and add to the beans
- Add tomato paste to mix well with the beans
- Add in paprika and mustard and stir for two minutes
- Add hot water to a level that creates a thick sauce
- Allow to cook for 12 minutes
- Add apple cider vinegar and salt to taste
- Cover and allow to cook for another 4 minutes

The recipe serves two. It takes several hours to prepare dried beans. Soak and cook beans after every few days to ensure you always have a ready batch when you want to cook. They can be refrigerated for a week. Beans are very nutritious. They contain soluble fibers. That quality enables them lower cholesterol in the body and control blood sugar levels. Refined sugars is the main cause of obesity. It is also linked to other lifestyle diseases such as cancer and heart disease. Therefore, it should be avoided.

Waldorf salad

It is a healthy salad containing low fat content. You can precook the rice so that you prepare the salad within a shorter time.

Ingredients

- Rice
- An apple
- A lemon
- One pepper of your choice
- 3 celery stalks
- Onion
- cup of walnuts

Process

- Cook the rice under low heat. Cook for around 45 minutes, until tender
- Chop pepper, celery and onion
- Chop walnuts
- Dice the apple and mix with freshly squeezed lemon juice
- After the rice is cooked, rinse using cold water
- Add olive oil

The recipe serves three people as a main meal. As a side dish, it serves up to six people. You can add a salad dressing for extra taste. If you want a light meal, replace the rice with a green salad.

Lightning Source UK Ltd.
Milton Keynes UK
UKHW020637090421
381714UK00011B/379

9 781802 170207